The Café Diet

Diet of the Roast Master

COFFEE | APPETITE | FOOD | EXERCISE

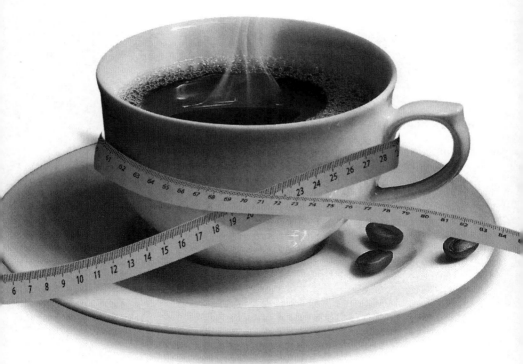

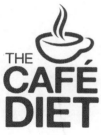

THE
CAFÉ
DIET

The Coffee Lovers Guide to Sustainable Fat Loss

Béla Csepregi

Disclaimer

This book is for informational purposes only and is in no way intended as medical advice, as a substitute for medical counseling, or as a treatment or cure for any disease or health condition nor should it be construed as such. This book is not meant to be used, nor should it be used, to diagnose or treat any medical condition. For diagnosis or treatment of any medical problem, consult your own physician.

The publisher and author are not responsible for any specific health or allergy needs that may require medical supervision and are not liable for any damages or negative consequences from any treatment, action, application or preparation, to any person reading or following the information in this book.

References are provided for informational purposes only and do not constitute endorsement of any websites or other sources. Readers should be aware that the websites listed in this book may change.

Dedicated

To my wife, Viki, who challenges me every day
with some sweet delights.
And
To my dad, who taught me to always stick to my principles.

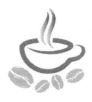

Acknowledgments

My heartfelt gratitude to the many people who assisted me in making this book a reality.

First of all, to *Roast Master Terry Davis,* who introduced me to the secrets of the coffee and the roasting process and who taught me how to roast and how to create perfect blends.

Thanks to *Cal Orey,* the bestselling author of several healing books, including *The Healing Powers of Coffees,* who encouraged me to pursue my book concept and helped me on my first steps toward publication.

Thank you to *Anja Thompson,* my favorite Kundali Yoga teacher, who kept her yoga classes going for months and accommodated my erratic schedule. Without her Kundalini Yoga classes, I would not be the same person.

I would like to say thank you to my employees, *Holly* and *Dimitry Erez* (Latitude 23.5 Coffee and Tea), for their never ending support and assistance in all my many experiments with the roaster and different types of coffee.

Contents

The Café Diet

Coffee…you either love it or you hate it. Sometimes you love it one way and hate it another. But there is no denying that coffee is the world's most popular beverage. My relationship with coffee was nothing special—probably something like yours is now—until I realized that it could be an essential element in my weight loss journey.

You see, I was born and raised in Europe, where "coffee culture" was like a religion. There were sects all over the place preaching the gospel of caffeine. You could not walk into a bistro or café without an extensive menu of strong, dark espressos, special roasts, and steamy, frothy extras to enjoy.

When I moved to the United States, I realized that things were different here. On the one hand, coffee was instant and necessary; on the other, it was a toasted delicacy that you could indulge in at your local coffee shop.

For me, my tango with coffee kicked off when I started working at a Floridian coffee roasting company. With beans from Kenya, Sumatra, India, Brazil, and Honduras, the possibilities were endless, and it ignited something inside me.

I found myself next to the roast master, and the rest, as they say, is history. I am now the roast master of that company, roasting several hundred pounds of coffee every day. I develop roasted coffees and blends for a living.

Coffee is a serious business, and while I have never been obese, I was certainly fat. My BMI was close to 28, and my cholesterol levels were climbing past 200. I would argue that being "overweight" and not obese makes it harder to lose that fat.

It is not like you look *that* bad or need to lose *that* much. This was always the reason, I guess, that the diets never worked for me. My doctor suggested the Mediterranean Diet, and I tried more than one weight loss program and loads of diet pills and smoothies until they were coming out of my ears. For some reason, the fat loss was always temporary.

Worse yet, I would gain back more fat after being on these diets. It was literally lose five pounds, gain seven. So I decided to combine my love for coffee and my need to lose weight. After carefully developing this system, I tested it on myself.

Turns out, coffee can be quite the lean, mean fat-loss accompaniment. I lost more than twenty-five pounds, and I have never felt better. That is what prompted me to develop the Café Diet. If hunger is your enemy, and your sluggish metabolism keeps ruining your fat loss efforts, you may want to try this easy-to-implement modern diet for the coffee-loving urbanite.

Health Warning!

Before engaging in any new type of weight loss diet or health plan, please consult your physician first, especially if you are taking prescribed medications or recovering from a surgical procedure. Ask your doctor about this plan if you are younger than 18, if you have an eating disorder, if you are pregnant or breastfeeding, or if you are a diabetic on insulin.

is For Caffeine: Wake Up and Smell The Coffee

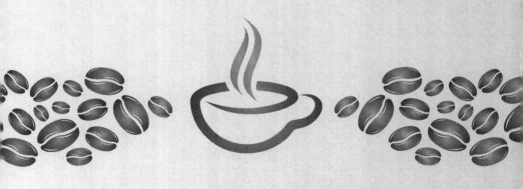

CHAPTER 1

Selected, Ground and Brewed: The Origins of Coffee

"Actually, this seems to be the basic need of the human heart in nearly every great crisis — a good hot cup of coffee."

ALEXANDER KING

Coffee and fat loss may seem like convenient friends, but there is real science behind the Café Diet. Of course, I only discovered this science once I had lost the bulk of my fat. Now I am a firm believer in guinea pigging myself for the sake of science.

If you are going to fall in love with this method of losing weight, I will need to start at the beginning. And like many beginnings, this one will take you way back—to a time when 1.6 billion cups of coffee was not being consumed globally each day.

What the Heck Is Coffee Anyway?

Coffee, as you know it, comes in a bag or a cup and is prepared in a variety of ways. But what the heck IS it? Chances are, you have never wandered into an orchard of coffee trees, and you have no idea how coffee even grows.

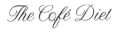

Coffee is a lot of different things to a lot of different people. Talk to the right people, and you will hear all about the miracle effects of coffee; talk to others and coffee might as well be a prisoner on the loose. Menace or miracle, it has captured the hearts and minds of people all over the world.

Coffee begins as a tree that—in the wild—could grow to more than 30 feet high. The tree is kept short and manageable, however, with rich dark green leaves that shine with a waxy luster. Red coffee cherries grow on the branches, and the flowers are soft and white.

Under the right circumstances, you would spot a white blossom coffee tree with green fruit and pinkish-red ripe fruit peeking out from under the leaves. A coffee farm will contain hundreds of trees and a league of refined workers to pick the ripe cherries.

Inside these coffee cherries are the beans, usually lying side-by-side in twos and nestled in an "envelope" that pros call the "parchment." Pickers sweep by each tree when the cherries are ripe to pick them. They are then whisked off to the coffee mill for processing.

In a coffee mill, the coffee beans are shucked from the cherries. Live, unroasted beans can last for months and may even become little coffee trees if water touches them.

After this long, amazing process, the coffee beans are processed, roasted, and packaged and arrive in your local grocery store. So coffee is the bean inside the fruit of the coffee tree.

A Scientific Breakdown of Your Favorite Blend

So how do you go from bean to your favorite coffee blend? There are two core types of coffee that are farmed and turned into your tasty morning cuppa. These are Coffea Arabica and Coffea. Both are scientific names for the types of beans used.

Coffea Arabica, or Arabica coffee as you may know it, is said to make the finest beans in the world. It makes sense then to take a closer look at what is inside those beans. I bet you can only name one thing, right? Caffeine.

Arabica coffee beans are typically made out of:

- **Caffeine:** A plant product found in coffee beans, this crystalline compound is a well-known nervous system stimulant.
- **Kahweol:** This is a molecule found in the Arabica plant that is making waves in the medical community because of its effects as an anti-inflammatory, anti-angiogenic compound that may also have beneficial effects on human bone structures.
- **Cafestol:** The other molecule in the coffee bean is cafestol, and studies have found it to be anti-carcinogenic, meaning that it has some use for fighting cancer in the human body. More studies are being conducted every day on these compounds.

Both Kahweol and Cafestol are diterpines, and they contribute to the unique flavor that you love in coffee. Add in an untold amount of natural antioxidants and the chemical make-up of a coffee bean is pretty clear.

Based on these three areas alone (caffeine, antioxidants, diterpines), coffee holds a very powerful list of health benefits for the coffee lover. Here are some main benefits:

- *Caffeine:* The pharmacologically active ingredient in the bean plays on your nervous system and enhances physical performance and mental alertness.
- *Antioxidants:* The compounds that your body cannot get enough of will help in cell defense and will actively deactivate oxidants.
- *Diterpines:* These are the compounds in coffee oil that have been found to assist as a protectant against some forms of cancer and various other diseases.

Coffea, or Robusta as it is known, is usually a lower quality coffee bean that contains higher levels of caffeine in it. Often both beans are blended together in different ways to produce different flavors and effects.

If you are a lover of quick-fix caffeine coffee, then you are a robusta type. For your gourmet flavors, you are looking at the higher quality Arabica blends, which are naturally lower in caffeine.

Science has proven that the humble bean (which is actually the seed of the coffee tree) is among the most fascinating of all fruit-based consumables in our natural world. We have only begun to study the properties of these beans!

The Roast Masters List of Coffee Variations

With Arabica and Robusta being the two main kinds of bean, nearly all coffee variations come from these delicious sources. But where the coffee grows and how it is roasted are two key elements in producing the long list of coffee variations available today.

- *Espresso:* Drunk in its natural state with a splash of boiling water, this strong, bitter coffee is a café staple across the world. Serve in shots.

- *Cappuccino:* A shot of coffee with steamed and frothed milk, topped with either nutmeg or chocolate, makes this an elegant café delight.

- *Café mocha:* Have a shot of coffee with steamed milk made with high quality hot chocolate and a dollop of cream. Dust the cream with chocolate powder.

- *Lattes:* Steam and foam milk then add to an equal amount of coffee and water. This is the cappuccino blend that focuses on a 50/50 split.

- *Americano:* A single or double shot of espresso with twice the amount of water in a traditional espresso cup, this is a straight shot of the good stuff.

- *Macchiato:* A single shot of espresso or two with a dollop of foamed milk makes the macchiato a little easier to drink without having to add in any milk.

- *Ristretto:* A concentrated shot of espresso presented as 22mls in the bottom of a coffee cup, it will wake up even the sleepiest people.

While these are the main variants of coffee, the "coffee culture" has become so widespread that today you can find anything from iced coffee to region-specific blends that are prepared in particular ways.

Heck, Starbucks alone gives you a variety of choices on how you get to drink a single espresso—the sky is the limit. From Café Cubano, Café Touba, Café Zorro and Decaf, to Black Tie, Green Eye, Mazagran, and Palazzo—the coffee industry is as rich and varied as any wine or aged alcoholic beverage.

As a roast master, I spend my days mixing and tasting coffee to get the right flavor, aroma, and lingering aftertaste. It is a very specific job that requires calm and focus. I fell in love with it immediately. So you can imagine my delight when coffee became the reason my fat started melting away.

I am not talking about a diet where you starve yourself and drink only coffee. I am talking about a diet that supports your modern, busy lifestyle and can help you shed those few extra pounds when you need to, quickly.

Best of all, coffee helps you keep them off. You do not need pills or special programs at all. The Café Diet is not meant to advocate the use of coffee to the exclusion of all reason and all other best practices. It is a system that I created that models fast fat loss on one of those stylish European street corners—the food, the coffee, the lifestyle.

The Epic Origin Story of Coffee

According to legend, the very first inkling that coffee may be excellent to consume was had by a goat herder named Kaldi, who noticed his goats getting frisky after eating the coffee berries off a nearby tree. These dancing goats in Ethiopia were just the beginning.

Soon tribes all over Africa were consuming the coffee beans in droves, and they preferred to roll it into little balls made of beans and fat that were protein-rich and gave them hours of excellent energy. Eventually, the energy bean made it across the sea to Arabia.

It was AD 1000 when the Arabians began roasting coffee to drink. By the 13th century Muslims were religiously drinking coffee and taking it all over the world: the Mediterranean, India, North Africa—all countries relatively close to each other.

During this time there was a total monopoly on coffee, as Arabia made every bean that left the country completely infertile. It was only after the 1600s that coffee beans made their escape, strapped to an Indian smuggler named Baba Budan.

Coffee, again, started to spread like wildfire. Eventually it moved from Turkey to Europe—Venice being the heart of the European coffee launch back then. Soon the Dutch found ways of getting coffee plants, and the first plantation in Europe opened for business.

Coffee trees were gifted to European aristocracy who kept them in their lush, royal gardens. A naval officer, Mr. Gabriel Mathieu de Clieu, wanted to take a clipping of the coffee tree to the new French colony in Martinique. On refusal, the bold young naval officer broke into the King's garden late one evening and got away with his clipping.

The bold de Clieu battled jealous passengers that tried to steal his clipping, a band of bloodthirsty pirates, and a storm that nearly had him at the bottom of Davie Jones' locker. Then the weather cleared up and water rations became scarce. He gave half of his water rations to his seedling.

With armed guards, the naval officer planted that tree in Martinique, creating 18 million trees and progeny that would eventually supply Latin America with its strains. Fast forward to 1727 and Brazil's super spy Lt Col. Francisco de Melo Palheta was sent to French Guiana, where he wooed the governor's wife and received a bouquet of seedlings for his trouble.

By 1800 Brazil had taken coffee from a rarity to the world's most in-demand drink—all thanks to the bravery of individuals who saw the potential in growing and farming this incredible crop. These days coffee is a billion dollar industry and is the second most traded commodity on earth, second only to oil.

The Etymology of Coffee: Shaping the World

So how did coffee end up changing and shaping the world? To get a clue about that, we have to take a closer look at the word coffee. Etymology is just a fancy way of referring to the study of the origin of a word and how the meaning has changed in history.

The real question is how did fat-rolled balls become the word coffee? Here is the process that this famous dark liquid invoked.

- The Arabic word for coffee was qahwah, which changed in Turkey to become kahveh, a word you can recognize as the basis for the English one.
- Other nations using it at the time called it café (French), caffe (Italian), koffie (Dutch), and eventually coffee (English).

Coffee as an English word first started appearing in literature when coffee was purchased by merchants returning from the Far East. In a famous book called "Rauwolf's Travels," Leonhard Rauwolf journeyed from Marseille in 1573 to Aleppo and returned in 1576.

He was the first European to ever mention coffee in literature and—as a matter of interest—was also a doctor of medicine and a world-renowned botanist. In "Rauwolf's Travel," coffee appears as the word "chaube" from the people in the city of Aleppo.

There were variations of the word among writers during the 16th century, but the first person to call it "coffee" was John Evelyn in 1637. He was a writer, a diarist, and a gardener who once again found the coffee tree a fascinating study.

Originally, the Arabic term for coffee, "qahwah," meant "wine," but as the meaning changed through language, development, and use, coffee came to mean a drink made from the evergreen coffee tree.

Today the definition has evolved to include various techniques for brewing coffee. I have no doubt that the meaning will continue to change as more methods and styles are unearthed. Coffee influenced history in so many ways.

The most important was the rise of business. Coffee houses in Europe became places to sit and enjoy the beverage while exchanging ideas. Everything from literature, newspapers, and great compositions from Bach and Beethoven were unleashed in coffee houses.

Thanks to the Boston Tea Party in 1773, Americans switched to coffee. This pulled Western civilization out from the thumb of beer and liquor and sparked a new kind of beverage for breakfast consumption—the humble cup of coffee.

Extremely Important People Who Love Coffee

Coffee is still in the process of improving the world by keeping influential people awake, alert, and ready for anything. Here are some extremely important people who love coffee so that you can understand how crucial it is in society today.

- Dan Lyons is the Editor in Chief of ReadWrite and a business genius. He has written for *Newsweek* and *Forbes* magazine. He confesses to loving the buzz of coffee and drinks four cups a day of Nescafe instant.

- Thomas Eliot, or TS Eliot as he is known, was one of the most influential American poets, playwrights, and writers of the

20th century. He famously said, "I have measured out my life with coffee spoons."

- Stieg Larsson's famous trilogy *Girl With a Dragon Tattoo* contained dozens of scenes where characters referenced coffee. The *New York Times* even mentioned how the book seemed to revolve around the making and consuming of the drink.

- The Netherlands has the highest coffee consumption per capita than any other country in the world, with 2.414 cups[1] per day. As an interesting side note, the Netherlands was recently ranked #1 out of all healthcare systems in the world.

- Balzac and Voltaire, two prominent figures of the French Revolution, were known to drink up to 50 cups of coffee a day because they loved it so much.

- Napoleon Bonaparte was a fierce coffee lover who asked for a spoon of coffee on his deathbed. On autopsy, they discovered ground coffee beans in his stomach.

- Howard Schultz loved coffee so much he founded a global empire around it. Starbucks is the most famous coffee franchise in America, based on specialty uses for this noble little beverage.

- Beethoven was one of the greatest composers that ever lived, and he liked his coffee ground into exactly 60 beans per cup— well over the normal amount of coffee you are supposed to drink per sitting.

- Thanks to Pope Clement VIII, coffee went from being "satanic" to being a beverage embraced by the church and therefore millions of Christians all over the world.

Coffee continues to be a mysterious and hugely influential beverage in modern society. You cannot deny that it has played a

---

1   Jamie Condliffe. The World's Biggest Coffee Drinkers, Visualized. http://gizmodo.com/the-worlds-biggest-coffee-drinkers-visualized-1502533056

role in developing the modern world and has helped progressive nations tap into the power of ideas for the benefit of mankind.

It is no wonder that this drink is revered by so many and used daily. But what if you could use coffee as a way of losing weight? What if coffee was the one thing that could help you keep all of that fat off your body? This is what the Café Diet suggests!

CHAPTER 2

The Miracle Healing Power of Coffee

"We want to do a lot of stuff; we're not in great shape. We didn't get a good night's sleep. We're a little depressed. Coffee solves all these problems in one delightful little cup."

JERRY SEINFELD

You have probably heard whispers about the "healing power" of coffee. Most people have experienced some of these powers—alertness, a faster metabolism—but science has proven that the humble coffee bean has a lot more to offer than we thought.

As I sidled along on my weight loss path, I started uncovering serious research about the many, many health benefits of this incredible seed.

The Real Elixir of Life: Your Favorite Java

Could coffee be the elixir of life? With large knowledge hubs like Harvard and the Mayo Clinic conducting volumes of studies on the bean, it just may be. Researchers from the National Institute of Health and the American Association of Retired Persons conducted a study on the relationship between drinking coffee and survival.

In a study[2] involving 173,141 women and 229,119 men that lasted more than 13 years, people between the ages of 50 and 71 in good health were studied. The study excluded cancer, stroke, and heart disease victims and included adjusted levels for smokers.

Their findings were pretty startling to say the least. From this huge cross section of people, they discovered that one cup of coffee a day lowered your risk of dying by 5% for women and 6% for men. Drink 4–5 cups a day and your risk plummets by 16% for women and 12% for men. Turns out five cups of java a day is truly the elixir of life.

The study discovered that coffee is jam packed with bioactive polyphenols—more than 1000 different types that impact human health. And while studies have also indicated caution against that long-standing energy boost caffeine, you can feel safe in the knowledge that drinking coffee is adding years onto your life.

With some 50% of Americans drinking three or more cups every day, I would say that is a great thing. Not to be outdone, a study was also published by Harvard Medical School in the Annals of Internal Medicine that confirmed these longevity benefits.

The study—made up of 84,201 women and 41,736 men— showed that risk of death was reduced by 7% in woman with one cup a day and 26% with four or more. Men benefitted slightly less than women but with similar results.

The overwhelming evidence indicated that coffee, in the right amounts, was extremely beneficial, while coffee in wrong amounts could have serious side effects and dangers. How little we know and understand about this incredible bean!

Wake Up to the Benefits of Antioxidants

As I mentioned before, coffee is made up of three things, one of which is a bucket load of antioxidants. Now you may remember that

---

2   Kirk Stokel. National Institutes of Health Discovers Protective Effects of Coffee. http://www.lef.org/magazine/mag2012/sep2012_Protective-Effects-Of-Coffee_01.htm

antioxidants are the body's personal guard against free radicals, those pesky by-products that are created from our food and environment. Coffee can help you combat the free radicals in your body!

Along with lengthening your life, the polyphenols found in coffee are bursting with other benefits. But I do not want to mislead you here, so let me give you the whole picture. Back in the '90s, antioxidants became the latest "marketing" trend, and food companies began using them to sell millions of units of frozen berries and green tea.

So many studies have falsely inflated results in order to sell products. I want to reiterate that while antioxidants in some forms (beta-carotene and vitamin C for example) can have conflicting data, polyphenols[3] are the kind of antioxidant found in the coffee bean, and there is plenty of evidence to back up their health benefits.

- Polyphenols are a type of antioxidant that supports the prevention of cardiovascular diseases, cancers, and osteoporosis.
- They have been found to protect against neurodegenerative diseases and chronic diseases of the immune system like diabetes.
- Polyphenols have beneficial effects on endothelial lining of blood vessels by increasing the availability of nitric acid and preventing the lipid oxidation underlying atherosclerosis.

The Western diet is shockingly lacking in natural sources of polyphenol antioxidants. But the latest research indicates that consuming these from a variety of sources has the best possible effect on the human body.

Combined, plant polyphenols will work to synergistically protect against heart disease, cancer, diabetes, vascular problems and other chronic, life-destroying diseases with no known side effects. Now, call me crazy, but an antioxidant that can do all that?

3   Laurie Barclay MD. The Disease-Fighting Power of Polyphenols, https://www.lef.org/magazine/mag2008/feb2008_The-Disease-Fighting-Power-Of-Polyphenols_01.htm

Surely by combining polyphenol enriched coffee in the right doses with polyphenol rich plant foods, your body will start destroying free radicals and rapidly boost your immune function, right? It did! This was one of the ways I managed to lose all of my fat.

It is also why the Café Diet focuses a *lot* on green leafy veggies and cocoa beans (yes, I said chocolate!). The multitude of polyphenol combinations in your diet will contribute to your body's return to its natural state—thin, healthy, and bursting with energy!

I am a coffee lover, so you can imagine my delight when my research suggested that I could lose fat fast and use coffee as the medium to do it. I daresay anyone looking to rapidly lose fat either long term or in short-term bursts can do it this way. It is actually very easy.

The Coffee Cure: Lowering Disease Potential

Some people have been calling it the "coffee cure," but we both know better than to believe that kind of hype. Marketers love to take real research and turn it into something else; something, I might say, that spreads all over the Internet and becomes "knowledge" in no time. Well, I have sorted through all of that trash to give you the truth.

And the truth is that coffee is no miracle cure. Like many other beneficial compounds, there are hundreds of reasons why certain studies turn out like they do. What coffee is, however—and this has been declared by modern science—is a disease protectant.

If you, or a family member, have a specific type of disease that runs in your family, you can and should use coffee daily to help lower your disease potential. That means including coffee in your life will help protect you against a disease you are likely to contract.

- Cancer protector – Coffee has been found to have potential cancer-fighting properties. Recently researchers found that coffee drinkers were 50% less likely to get liver cancer than people that did not drink coffee. Reductions in rectal, breast, and colon cancer have also been widely documented.

- Diabetes protector – People that drink lots of coffee are less likely to contract diabetes as compared to light drinkers or non-drinkers. Coffee can lower blood sugar, and it increases metabolism, which keeps diabetes away.
- Blood pressure was previously thought to be negatively affected by coffee, though recent studies have shown that it does not, in fact, increase your risk for high blood pressure at all.
- Parkinson's disease protector – Coffee has been found to protect men, but not women, from this disease. Women can thank estrogen for the variance.

A USF study[4] showed that a "mystery" ingredient in coffee was responsible for countering Alzheimer's disease by improving memory in mice. The study mentions how this "unknown" ingredient combines with the caffeine and boosts blood levels, a critical growth factor when fighting off dementia and Alzheimer's.

USF researchers went on to mention that drinking coffee later in life can, in fact, as the data suggests, protect against these diseases. So you see, even coffee has an untold treasure trove of health benefits that we are only now coming to understand.

As you continue to read about the incredible benefits of coffee, keep in mind that this is to prepare you for using this substance correctly, in a diet that will help you lose fat and gain health.

Bean There Done That: Coffee and Stress

You might be thinking—but if coffee is so good at helping people gain health and lose fat, why is obesity a problem in this "coffee culture" age? I thought about this one long and hard, but sometimes the simplest answers are the best ones.

---

4   USF Health News Archives. USF study: Mystery ingredient in coffee boosts protection against Alzheimer's disease. http://hscweb3.hsc.usf.edu/health/now/?p=19816

Stress—it is the silent killer that has been plaguing the Western world for far too long now. You may have heard some negative things about how coffee raises your stress levels, and they are totally true. Caffeine is a nervous system stimulant, and it is widely abused by people needing to stay up late, work harder, and get ahead in life.

But there is a medical connection here that we are not seeing. Stress is the one thing that harms your health nearly all the time. It also makes you fat. With high levels of cortisol in your body, your waist to hip ratio will certainly increase.

Cortisol is a stress hormone that is released in the human body via the adrenal glands. It causes anxiety, sleep issues, cravings, and a host of other negative effects[5] in your body.

Lack of sleep and higher stress levels keep cortisol high in your body. You cannot lose weight when your cortisol levels are off the charts! Fact! And caffeine in coffee stimulates the secretion of cortisol in the human body, according to NIH Public Access. So why would you drink coffee if it aggravates your cortisol levels?

I thought about it long and hard. How was I going to use coffee to lose fat when the research indicated that coffee would make me *more* stressed and *less* likely to lose any fat. The only answer was to take a hard look at my existing cortisol levels.

Western civilization glorifies stress and being busy, even though it kills everyone. Only recently have people begun to actively practice and control their daily cortisol levels. If you can learn to do that, you can drink coffee at the right time—and it *will* help you lose weight.

I know because I did it. Real fat loss happened for me when I began to care about the cortisol levels in my body. I discovered that I was drinking coffee at the wrong times and flooding my body with caffeine—which resulted in a caffeine tolerance.

---

5   Lissa, Rankin, 10 Signs You Have Way Too Much Cortisol, http://lissarankin.com/10-signs-you-have-way-too-much-cortisol

Because of this, I drank more and more coffee—and my cortisol levels were consistently high. It is one of the reasons why my cholesterol levels were so off the charts! Too much cortisol and you are in the heart disease conga line. No one gets out alive.

So you could say I have been there and done that. I am an advocate of using coffee and a collaborative diet—but only if you understand that stress, and cortisol, will ruin the method. You cannot lose fat when your body is in overdrive from high cortisol levels. You must first learn to monitor them then coffee will become your best friend again.

The New Rules of Mental Acuity: Coffee Wins!

Boy oh boy, I will never forget the morning I woke up and downed four cups of coffee in a row and *still* did not feel awake. There is a reason for this you know. Your body creates its own version of caffeine in the morning between 8 and 9 a.m. for most people.

When you march into the kitchen, desperate to feel awake, your body is already trying to get you there. Little do you know that flooding your body with coffee is doing the opposite—it is making it harder for you to wake up. All you feel is the crash for the rest of the day. This is the coffee-cortisol cycle, and it needs to end.

Once it has ended, you can finally wake up refreshed once more. Let's be honest, you drink coffee because you want that boost in mental acuity and performance right away. It is ironic that your sleep cycles and cortisol take that away from you.

A recent report[6] concluded that caffeine effectiveness is directly related to when you consume it because of your body's cortisol cycle!

But this does not mean that you can never enjoy the huge mental benefits of caffeine ever again. With this diet, you will learn how to

---

6   Lizette Borreli, What's the Best Time to Drink Coffee? The House Matters Because Cortisol Cycle Influences Caffeine Effectiveness, http://www.medicaldaily.com/whats-best-time-drink-coffee-hour-matters-because-cortisol-cycle-influences-caffeine-effectiveness

do just that. Here is what coffee can do for your mental performance and memory when you use it correctly in your diet.

- *Low* doses of caffeine improve mental performance. The equivalent of two cups of high quality coffee (Arabica) causes mood elevation and alertness. It has also been found to improve working memory.
- *High* doses of caffeine cause sensory overload. Too much coffee during the day and you will suffer from anxiety attacks, insomnia, and mood issues.

These are the two most basic rules of mental acuity when you drink coffee. You do not want to go for loads of caffeine, because you will build up a tolerance and your cortisol levels will skyrocket, resulting in horrible side effects.

WARNING! Some people have an intolerance to caffeine,[7] in which case this diet is not recommended. Rapid heart rate, sleep disturbances, digestive upsets, and jitters are all plain signs of caffeine intolerance.

Consume small amounts of coffee at the right time, and you can enjoy that incredible "rush" of energy, alertness, and concentration that can only come from low dose caffeine and high quality beans. After all, coffee has long been used as medicine in different cultures; it is, above all, a very specific compound.

Caffeine is considered to be one of the safest kinds of stimulant that you can take. Used in low, accurate doses, it can facilitate fat loss. But of course, this all depends on your diet, your stress levels, and your lifestyle.

For now, all you need to know is that coffee is the greatest mental and physical performance enhancer there is—if you take the trouble to learn how to use it. I am going to show you how and more in the

7   Signs and Symptoms of Caffeine Intolerance, http://www.livestrong.com/article/538019-signs-symptoms-of-caffeine-intolerance/

Café Diet. You will be shedding those pounds in no time, with this safe, delicious, and natural stimulant from the earth.

The Real Bad Wrap: Coffee Vs. Sugar

You have probably read some disturbing things about coffee online about how it makes you gain weight, makes you get moody, and pushes you into a cycle of ill health. I would like to be the first to say that these are mostly lies directed at coffee when the real culprit is...sugar.

Most people in the Western world take their coffee with milk, cream, and lots of sugar. While this turns a great drink into an outstanding one, it also ruins all the health benefits of coffee. Sugar is no fat loss supplement, and recent studies have determined that it may be the main reason why there is such a surge in chronic diseases in the world.

Drinking coffee with sugar is kind of like eating an apple that has been dipped in maple syrup—it is sweet, but the negative effects of the sugar have demolished any positive effects that the original source might have had. So it is with coffee. Sugar is its worst enemy.

- Sugar is highly addictive, leading to the overuse of coffee and the current obesity epidemic in America.
- Sugar has been found to suppress your immune system function, causing metabolic disease, diabetes, and other chronic digestive disease.
- Sugar leads to all kinds of nutrient deficiency and worse—the more you eat it, the more you want it—until eventually you are only eating different forms of sugar. Look at the modern diet of carbohydrates (sugars), junk food (sugar), processed food (sugar), sweets (sugar), and some kinds of chocolate (sugar).
- Sugar increases heart disease, Alzheimer's, dementia, cancer, and several of the most widespread and threatening modern illnesses.

It is safe to say that sugar has given coffee a bad rap. It is even worse when you consider the confusion behind sugar—and how it is in *everything* these days. Literally everything from baby food, to sodas, sauces, soups, condiments, and all packaged meats contain sugar.

You could be eating loads of sugar every day and not even know it. My advice would be to cut down on your sugar intake as much as possible or just cut it out completely.

Just to let this sink in a bit—sugar was recently proclaimed more lethal than cocaine on the addiction scale. Robert Lustig, a doctor apart, has been calling for new laws regulating sugar in food. These laws are coming, and it is best to understand them.

So when I speak about coffee, I am not talking about the deathly sweet "coffee and three spoons" version. I am talking about pure, rich, delicious coffee, with a splash of milk, half and half, or black— or a hint of honey for sweetness.

CHAPTER 3

Practical Fat Loss With Aromatic Coffee

"It is inhumane, in my opinion, to force people who have a genuine medical need for coffee to wait in line behind people who apparently view it as some kind of recreational activity."

DAVE BARRY

I mentioned that there are two main types of coffee bean, coffea Arabica and coffea robusta. Coffea Arabica is usually the higher quality bean with the most aromatic scents and flavors. It is also low caffeine, which suits our dietary purposes.

Your choice of coffee matters because no two blends are created equally. You want to specifically target rich, full-flavored roasts made from low-caffeine Arabica. That way, you can apply your blends to your practical fat loss regimen.

The Science of When to Drink Coffee: Portion Control

Every living person in the world has something called a circadian clock. This is your 24-hour hormonal cycle that naturally occurs in the body. It works off your internal rhythm and tells you when to wake up, to eat, or to exercise for example.

Your body also produces cortisol, which is the stress hormone that wakes you up. You might recall I mentioned it is impossible to lose fat while you are full of cortisol. That said, your body produces cortisol at peak times between 8 and 9 a.m.

Before you ever take that first sip of morning coffee, your body has already caffeinated itself. Drinking more coffee only leads to overload, and it will completely erase that "buzzed" feeling you are supposed to get from coffee.

To gain control of your coffee use for fat loss, you need to get a handle on two things: cortisol times and portion control. If you can control the amount of caffeine you drink and when you drink it, you can use the powers of caffeine for positive fat loss.

- Coffee portions! There is no such thing as an "average" amount of caffeine in your coffee. You have to check and make sure that you are not consuming much more than 300–400 milligrams every day. Sometimes that is one cup of coffee from your local coffee shop; sometimes it is four cups of coffee from your instant home brand.

- Women on birth control pills metabolize caffeine twice as slowly—so the impact of the caffeine hits them twice as hard. Make a note of that!

- Some people metabolize coffee slower than others; you need to work out what your body is telling you. The safe way is to never go above 400 milligrams per day.

- Keep in mind that caffeine can disguise itself in other food sources, so get into the habit of reading food labels and avoiding high caffeine foods and drinks.

- The when is simple—studies[8] suggest that you should not drink coffee as soon as you wake up. Wait until 9:30–11:30 for your

8   Fries, E, L Dettenborn, The Cortisol Awakening Response (CAR): Facts and Future Directions, http://www.ncbi.nlm.nih.gov/pubmed/18854200

first cup of java. Then wait until 12:00–1:00 for more. This is a loose guideline as long as you track how many cups you are having a day. Let's face it; coffee in the morning is critical!

Metabolism Booster: 10 Powerful Fat-Loss Coffee Recipes

If you are able to stick to the times that science suggests our bodies will maximize the use of caffeine in our coffee, you can use it as a metabolism booster. The faster your metabolism goes, the more fat you will burn.

1. *Espresso*: Force a small amount of nearly boiling water under pressure through finely ground coffee beans. Gold foam should form on the surface. Drink it black, with no sugar or a dash of half and half.

2. *Cappuccino*: Add equal parts of espresso, steamed milk, and milk froth for this delicious French favorite. Sprinkle with unsweetened cocoa powder.

3. *Americano*: This is a single shot of espresso mixed into a cup of boiling water. Add milk to taste, although a splash is the traditional method. Add stevia instead of sugar.

4. *Caffe Latte*: A single shot of espresso with three parts steamed milk, it is rich and creamy and deserves a sprinkling of cocoa on the top.

5. *Café Mocha*: Also called a Mochachino, this is a basic caffe latte or cappuccino with added cocoa powder or chocolate syrup. Avoid the syrup versions, and add stevia to taste.

6. *Café au Lait*: Instead of espresso, simply blend brewed coffee in a cup with steamed milk in equal parts.

7. *Espresso Con Panna*: Enjoy a wonderful shot of espresso with a large dollop of fresh whipped cream and a sprinkling of cocoa powder on top.

8. *Red Eye*: A shot of espresso with a normal instant blend on top, this can be taken if you only plan on having one cup in the morning.
9. *Cafe Breve*: This is a single shot of espresso with steamed half and half and a nice topping of frothy milk foam dusted with cocoa.
10. *Just Black*: Break out your favorite instant brand, and steep a teaspoon of coffee in boiling water. Drink in a ceramic cup, no sugar, no milk. Just black.

You may note that cream and milk froth are still used in these recipes, and for good reason. I did not have to cut out cream or milk in my diet. In fact, I found that the less sugar I ate and the more cream I consumed, the more the fat fell off me.

As it turns out, you can have cream every day if that is what you like. When your diet is not full of sugar, there are zero health risks to having cream, and it does not make you put on weight as previously thought!

Green Beans of Delight: Melting Belly Fat

Recent studies have indicated that green coffee bean supplements make people drop a significant percentage of their body fat when taken daily. The study was conducted at the University of Scranton in Pennsylvania with 16 obese people over 22 weeks.

No eating habits or exercise changes were allowed. It was just them and the good old green beans. The study found that participants lost 17 pounds on average. That is a total weight loss of 10% and a total fat loss of 16%!

So what makes green coffee beans so great at melting fat? It cannot be the caffeine, or these effects would be seen all over the globe. Scientists discovered it was due to a compound called chlorogenic acid.

The bad news is that roasted coffee breaks down chlorogenic acid, which means your average cuppa will not have these fat-melting properties. With zero side effects and clinical evidence that these coffee beans cause fat loss, why would you not take them?

Because the study was very small, and research on green coffee beans is just starting out. Even Dr. Oz did his own study of 100 women on green coffee beans and found that on average the participants in his unqualified study lost two pounds on the supplement.

Science is still trying to catch up to the potential for coffee to make people lose fat. You can turn the green beans into a drink like their roasted brethren, but it is very bitter. The active ingredient in green coffee beans is said to reduce blood pressure and assist the body in blood sugar and metabolic function.

Until further studies are done, I want to say this. I have tried green coffee, and it is not my favorite to drink. But I did feel healthier when I was drinking it. I see no harm at all in adding these little capsule supplements to your diet if you want a helping hand.

Just make sure that you check on the caffeine levels as well. The last thing you want is to be taking caffeine in capsule form while drinking coffee. This will lead to heart palpitations and all sorts of unpleasant side effects that you can avoid.

Why put green coffee beans into the book if I do not use them? It *is* the Café Diet, is it not? I want to tell you all about the world of coffee and fat loss, even the shady bits. You can choose to believe the studies and Dr. Oz, or you can leave this part out.

Personally, I find that my normal coffee routines and eating plans do enough for me. But I would never suggest cutting out green coffee, because there are not enough studies on it yet. For all we know, chlorogenic acid may just be the fat loss miracle is claims to be!

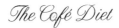

Avoiding Dehydration Risk: H2O Supplementation

Coffee is perhaps the most famous diuretic in the world. As soon as you have had a cup, off you go to find the nearest facilities. But moderate levels of caffeine do not cause dehydration, a study has recently found.

The Institute for Scientific Information on Coffee funded the study that involved 50 men. They each drank four mugs of black coffee or four mugs of water a day for three days. Then after a 10-day period, the men switched—one group drinking coffee, the other water.

The participant's hydration status was measured using their total body water and body mass. There were no significant differences. That said, a paper was assembled by a scientist from the University of Connecticut.

His review of 10 previous studies indicated an 84% retention of the total volume of coffee ingested, while water only had an 81% retention rate. So why do so many health professionals suggest drinking more water when people consume coffee?

Misinformation: Our modern diet has left many of us avoiding water and drinking sodas, teas, coffee, and other drinks instead. We have become so far removed from our habit of drinking lots of water that the only thing that compares is coffee.

Granted, a high caffeine cup of java *will* cause your metabolism to speed up. So dehydration can in fact occur with coffee abuse. Too much caffeine and you could find yourself very thirsty indeed.

While you are transitioning from sugar-loaded beverages to coffee, consider supplementing your water intake. It will help you detox, and it will make sure that you avoid any dehydration, which will reduce your fat loss progress.

If your body thinks it is dehydrated, it will store water. Most of us live in a perpetual state of dehydration, which is the real enemy here. Along with your excellent 3–5 cups of coffee a day, add on the equivalent for water.

This will get your body back into a state of hydration, which will jumpstart your metabolism along with the low levels of caffeine. You will be feeling like a million bucks by the end of your first month. I say month because sugar detox will make you feel terrible for at least two weeks. You should try to eliminate the sugar or try to use the least amount possible.

One Cup a Day: The Process of Caffeine Induced Fat Loss

Caffeine is a stimulant, but it is also a low level psychoactive. Caffeine has been used in weight loss supplements for as long as they have been around. It is important to understand how caffeine plays on the human body and mind.

Scientific research has told us that caffeine stimulates the central nervous system, which sends signals to your fat cells and tells them to break down. Caffeine increases the level of epinephrine in our blood, which is a hormone that causes an adrenaline response.

When epinephrine travels through your blood and into your fatty tissue, it gives off signals that cause the fat to be released into the blood. Once in free fatty acid form, the body can metabolize the fat or dispose of it.

Then there are the excellent metabolic reactions that caffeine causes. Our resting metabolic rate is affected—meaning that our metabolisms are kicked into high gear when we consume caffeine. Studies have shown that caffeine increases your resting metabolic rate by as much as 11%. An increase in metabolism is a direct result of the fat burning process.

If you are fairly lean, some studies support the evidence that you can lose as much as 29% of your fat after consuming caffeine on a regular basis. Obese people can lose 10%. The younger you are, the more caffeine works to your benefit.

So having at least one cup of coffee a day can bring you all of these amazing caffeine benefits. And I have not even mentioned how you can use caffeine to improve your physical performance just yet.

Exercise performance is easily increased with the use of caffeine by some 11–12%.[9] Drinking coffee before exercising will put your body into a fat burning state, which will further propel your metabolism, resulting in a boost in fat loss.

So you see, caffeine can be good, and it can be bad. Bad because people tend to overuse it and then burn out or give themselves serious side effects. Worst case scenario is that you are tweaking every day and have no fat loss to show for it.

But if you use caffeine responsibly, in its natural form (coffee!) and as part of a complete, fat-burning diet, I have to say that it is the best way to burn fat I have *ever* used. Improve your resting metabolic rate, and burn more fat before you exercise.

I will speak more about coffee and exercise later on, but for now, I want you to understand that it is caffeine that is the major fat-burning agent in coffee. But it is not the only one! As science has admitted time and time again, coffee is still largely an enigma.

Supporting Your Goals: Good Guy Coffee Beans

Another fad diet—you may be thinking—but it is not. The Café Diet is not a lifestyle plan or a long-term weight loss model. It is based on science, on my physical evidence, and on the many people I have helped burn fat with coffee.

Most of all, coffee is a wonderful, natural tool to support a healthy, fat burning diet. Remember I spoke about the added benefits of eating different types of polyphenols? That is just one reason. When you combine caffeine in coffee—with the right food—something

---

9   Kris Gunnars. Can Coffee Increase Your Metabolism and Help You Burn Fat? http://authoritynutrition.com/coffee-increase-metabolism/

magic happens. The fat around your belly, in particular, melts off!

Caffeine is also a natural appetite suppressant, which means that when you are going through that insane sugar detox, you will not be as hungry if you drink coffee. I have found it is best to add "detox periods" into your coffee diet.

A short two-week cycle is all it takes to lose those extra pounds. Even though I sound like a weight loss infomercial, the truth stands. I have tried those other fad diets, and they were always impossible to stick to. The hunger was too bad.

With the Café Diet, you are able to better quit your addiction to sugar with the help of a fat-burning natural compound that also suppresses appetite and invigorates your mind enough to stick to your diet! Like I said earlier, it is the simple solutions that often work the best.

These days I think of caffeine as "good guy coffee" because in all of my fat loss efforts it has been there, supporting me. It was very difficult to not overuse coffee in my position as a roast master—but I did. I took control of my portions, my methods, and my drinking times.

If you can do the same, I can promise you that this little diet secret will help you lose that fat when you need to. Have a wedding coming up? The Café Diet! Have to look good in a school reunion tux? The Café Diet?

Like the coffee itself, it is a quick way to speed up your fat loss efforts. Now that you understand the hype behind coffee and the huge benefits that it can give you, I will go through the rest of the diet with you.

I recently went in for a blood test to check my sugar levels. Before I started using the Café Diet, my fasting blood sugar levels sat at 98. The danger zone for pre-diabetes is between 100 and 125. That day my fasting blood sugar level was 71, with 70 being at the bottom of the normal range.

This is conclusive proof that the intermittent fasting helped repair my insulin sensitivity to create normal blood sugar levels. There are studies[10] that support my own guinea pig work on low carb, intermittent fasting diets being beneficial for diabetics! Even though I have a bottom end blood sugar level, I can still work a highly physical job, and I never feel dizzy or ill.

Coffee has also recently been found to reduce the risk of colon cancer by 30%[11] along with lowering the risk for other cancers like prostate and breast and skin cancer.

Whether you need to lose all of your fat or just a few key pounds—or you just want to be healthier—you can scale and adjust this diet as needed. The trick is to steer clear of sugar, to manage your food intake, and to support your fat loss goals with a delicious selection of fine Arabica coffee blends.

---

10 New Study: A Low-Carb Diet and Intermittent Fasting Beneficial for Diabetics, http://www.dietdoctor.com/new-study-low-carb-diet-intermittent-fasting-beneficial-diabetics

11 Racheal Rettner, Drinking Coffee May Cut Risk of Colon Cancer, http://www.livescience.com/44688-drinking-coffee-may-cut-risk-of-colon-cancer.html

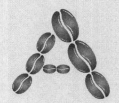

Is for Appetite: Time for a Coffee Break

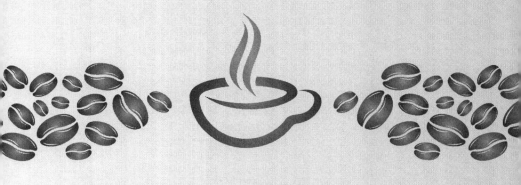

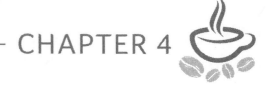

CHAPTER 4

Principles of Using Coffee for Fat Loss

*"It doesn't matter where you're from—or how you feel...
There's always peace in a strong cup of coffee."*

GABRIEL BÁ

In section II of the Café Diet, I will launch into the finer principles of how coffee can help you lose fat. Practical application is what matters in this chapter, and I am going to share with you a lot of great information I picked up during my time testing out different methods.

Your appetite and learning to control it is paramount to your success with this innovative diet. If you can follow these basic principles, I promise you that you will experience the thrill of shedding weight with very little physical effort.

The Real Calories in Coffee: Cutting Them Out

As I have established, coffee is surprisingly good for the human body. Why then has it received such terrible reviews over the past few decades? I remember reading all about "reducing your coffee intake" a few years ago because it makes you fat.

Headlines focused on "sabotaging diets" with coffee and on all the negative effects of over-using caffeine. As it turns out, the weight loss community was not targeting the coffee; they were targeting the calories in coffee. And the calories in coffee come directly from the "extras" that have been added to make the coffee taste better.

I am referring to sugar, cream, milk, and flavorants of course. So using coffee to facilitate fat loss is only possible once you understand that the real calories in coffee come from all the ingredients that are not coffee. That is why the following matters:

- The type of coffee that you drink matters. A cup of full bodied Arabica is low caffeine, has no fat, and has only two to four calories when consumed without any extras.

- The way you drink your coffee matters. A cup of coffee with two sugars shoots up to 34 calories. Add milk, and you are looking at 52 calories. Add cream, and your four-calorie cup of coffee now holds a whopping 103 calories.

- Fast food coffee is even worse because it contains ice cream, cream, and sugar, which can skyrocket the calorie range to 400–630 calories!

Everyone knows that to lose fat you have to think about the calories that you are consuming. So while you may love your sugar-infused coffee, it *is* harming your fat loss goals. To reverse this situation, remove the sugar from your coffee and only use cream occasionally.

If you love sweet coffee with milk, simply substitute the sugar for a small teaspoon of natural raw honey. Each cup is round about 36 calories, which is perfect. Even better, however, is no sweetener at all for a neat coffee and milk experience at 22 calories.

The Buzz: Understanding What Happens in Your Body

Coffee has seen some bad press because of caffeine abuse, but caffeine is not unique to coffee at all. In fact, over 60 plants contain caffeine—including tea, cacao, and kola nuts. Then you still have the plethora of man-made caffeine products to contend with.

According to an Ohio study, one in five students (7th, 8th, and 9th graders) consume more than 100mg[12] of caffeine every day. In fact, the average American consumes about 230mg[13] a day, which is the equivalent of about two cups of coffee. You should never exceed 400mg, or four 16-ounce cups of coffee, as you are likely to experience side effects of caffeine overdose.

So what happens inside your body when you consume a cup of coffee? In other words, how do you get the buzz that everyone loves so much from coffee? This is how:

- After 10 minutes of drinking your cup of coffee, the caffeine enters your bloodstream and increases your heart rate. Your blood pressure begins to rise.

- After 20 minutes you begin to feel more awake and more alert. Increased concentration and the ability to solve problems happens with greater ease. This can continue for up to four hours after consuming coffee.

- After 30 minutes, increases in the concentration of serotonin improve your motor neuron activity, which means that your muscles become more efficient. Adrenaline floods your body and fights off fatigue while boosting your energy levels.

- After four hours of consuming just 50mg of coffee, your body increases energy expenditure—even when you are sitting down. That means you can sit and burn fat more efficiently when you are doing nothing.

---

12 Medicines in my Home: Caffeine and Your Body, http://www.fda.gov/downloads/drugs/resourcesforyou/consumers/buyingusingmedicinesafely/understandingover-the-countermedicines/ucm205286.pdf
13 Caffeine, http://www.dorchesterhealth.org/caffeine.htm

- After six hours, feelings of contentment and inertia take over as your anxiety naturally decreases.

Improved performance and mental acuity are excellent fat loss accompaniments. The buzz you feel from coffee is literally the adrenaline and serotonin combining to make you feel more energized than before.

Because caffeine acts on your central nervous system, you have to be aware that drinking too much coffee will induce negative side effects. In fact, the latest research[14] indicates that you should never drink more than 28 cups of coffee per week, or four a day.

The caffeine content is really to blame, however. You could have six cups of low caffeine coffee a day and still be fine. The key is to remember that coffee used in the right doses will facilitate a boost in your metabolism, and you will accelerate your fat loss.

How to Harness Caffeine for Appetite Control

Caffeine used in the right way can be an incredible appetite suppressant. I discovered this while suffering through pretty severe hunger issues when I began to lose fat and detox off sugar. It was hard, but the coffee helped.

According to Duke University,[15] caffeine can be used to mask hunger because it acts as a stimulant in your body. The debate has been raging for quite some time, with many firsthand reports (like mine) of people feeling less hungry when they sip on coffee during the day.

There is also an ongoing study from Griffith University[16] to test how coffee affects the human appetite. Some participants drink

---

14   Maria Godoy, How Many Cups of Coffee Per Day Are Too Many?, http://www.npr.org/blogs/thesalt/2013/08/17/212710767/how-many-cups-of-coffee-per-day-is-too-many

15   Caffeine, https://studentaffairs.duke.edu/studenthealth/nutrition/nutrition-resources-information/caffeine

16   Coffee and Weight Control: How Coffee Impacts Appetite and Metabolism, http://cathe.com/coffee-and-weight-control-how-coffee-impacts-appetite-and-metabolism

a cup of joe in the early morning then again later that morning. Others drink all sorts of caffeinated beverages.

The results so far are consistent; participants feel less hungry and have a greater feeling of satiety after drinking coffee. The great news is that as you are using coffee to reduce your hunger cravings, it is also boosting your metabolism by 3–4%.

To get the most out of your caffeine fix in your coffee, you should be drinking no more than three cups of coffee a day. The first and second cup should be consumed in the morning and then one again at lunch time.

It works best once you have detoxed off sugar. Sugar is the one thing that can corrupt your fat loss progress with coffee. That is because sugar throws off your body's ability to regulate hunger correctly—which leaves it in a permanent state of starvation.

If you have a sweet tooth and are prone to eating a lot of sugary foods and carb-based foods, you most likely suffer from extreme hunger pains all the time. These are not natural. Hunger is supposed to be a gentle nudge towards food, a non-painful alarm bell caused by your body's internal systems.

What sugar does is corrupt your hormones, which leads your body to believe that it is existing in a perpetual state of hunger. If your stomach hurts like crazy when you are hungry, there is every chance that sugar has messed up your body's natural hormone production.

The Dangers of Coffee Abuse: Comfort Eating

Coffee, as wonderful and invigorating as it is, still contains caffeine, which is a highly addictive and very dangerous drug. In recent years coffee consumption has increased from an average of 3.3 cups per person to 4.6 cups per person in the 18–24 age range.[17]

---

17 Tracey Roizman, What Are the Dangers of Coffee Abuse, http://healthyeating. sfgate.com/dangers-coffee-abuse-1658.html

No doubt that it is our stressful, busy, and hectic lifestyles that are to blame. Using a substance to keep yourself alert, focused, and awake is still drugging—whether it is socially acceptable or not. But overusing coffee leads to significant detrimental side effects that you cannot afford to deal with.

- Caffeine, a central nervous system stimulant, when combined with sugar, is a lethal combination. This is because sugar is also incredibly addictive, more so than caffeine and potentially more than other, illegal drugs. Sugar cravings are real, and reaching for a cup of coffee to satisfy them will lead to comfort eating.
- Comfort eating happens when your body is exhausted and your moods are low. You feel depressed or sad or have a severe lack of energy from overusing coffee—so you drink more sugar-laden coffee to try and cure it. This triggers hunger for sugar-rich foods, sweets, fast food, and carbohydrates that make you fat.

The really crazy thing is that being tired and hungry all the time increases your stress levels to the point where your cortisol levels are sky high. As I mentioned before, cortisol suppresses immunity, it causes your muscles to break down, and it increases your visceral abdominal fat. It is a vicious cycle that all begins with coffee addiction.

And coffee addiction comes from not regulating how much coffee you put into your body or not being aware of how much caffeine is in coffee that you drink. Even when you go out to eat, you have the right to ask your local coffee shop how much caffeine is in their coffee.

You should do this for a few reasons; namely, because coffee houses tend to load their coffee with caffeine because it sells more beverages. Better yet, it sells all of those tasty doughnuts, hotdogs, and other carbohydrates that they are selling.

Comfort eating is a modern phenomenon that is ruining the health of people all over America and contributing to the obesity epidemic. It is short sighted to believe that the coffee–sugar partnership is not at least somewhat to blame.

You need to be on your guard against escalating your coffee intake and contributing to that vicious cycle. Believe me, if you do not watch out, your coffee intake will increase and along with it, your waist line. It is a delicate balance but one that works very well.

The Correct Doses at the Right Time

Enjoying coffee is something that comes naturally, but what does not come naturally are the imposed times and circumstances that you need to learn about when using coffee to lose fat. The correct doses at the right times will accelerate your fat loss efforts, like they did to mine.

Neuroscientists conducted tests and determined that the best time to drink coffee is, in fact, between 9:30 and 11:30 a.m.[18] While this is not an ironclad rule, if you suffer from extreme fatigue, you may want to try it out to regulate your cortisol levels.

If you cannot stick to those guidelines, then you only have to wait an hour until enjoying your first cup of coffee. I usually get up, mess around a bit, and then as the hour approaches, enjoy my first cup. This gives me the energy I need to face the day and to do it in a way that promotes the diet that is helping me lose weight.

While you are regulating your coffee intake, it is important to make sure that you do not use caffeine in other products. Things like energy drinks and certain types of food can contain large amounts of caffeine, which would trigger the negative side effects.

---

18   Richard Gray, Best Time to Drink a Cup of Coffee: 10:30am, http://www.telegraph.co.uk/news/newstopics/howaboutthat/10430303/Best-time-to-drink-a-cup-of-coffee-10.30am.html

Coffee is also about circumstances, and it can be used in two very useful ways. Both of these methods saved me on more than one occasion when I was on the diet.

- Just before exercising I would have a cup of coffee. This is because coffee is one of the world's best and safest ergogenic aids. It enhances performance and helps you train faster, harder, and longer. There are over 74 different studies[19] on the use of caffeine in exercise and sport. The overwhelming conclusion is that caffeine makes physical exercise easier, sometimes by as much as 12%.

- If you are feeling unmotivated about your diet or are hungry, drink a cup of coffee. This is because of caffeine's ability to reduce hunger pain and its instant focus effect. There is nothing worse than feeling tired, hungry, and unmotivated. Coffee can bring you back from choosing to phone the food delivery service.

Please understand that coffee varies from person to person. Some people only need a quarter of a cup, and they are buzzing for hours. All of the doses recommended here should be tested according to your own physiology.

You can read all of the studies in the world and still never arrive at a dose that perfectly suits your body, because of your genetics! Keep calm, and start the testing process slowly. You will be coming off the effects of sugar, which will be tough.

The best advice I can give you is to document when the best time to drink coffee is for you. It might be 5 a.m. in the morning or 2 p.m. in the afternoon. It all depends on your unique stress levels, metabolism, and chemical makeup.

---

19   Nancy Clark, The Facts About Caffeine and Athletic Performance, http://www. active.com/articles/the-facts-about-caffeine-and-athletic-performance

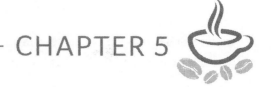

The Pervasiveness of Coffee in Society

"The powers of a man's mind are directly proportioned to the quantity of coffee he drinks."
JAMES MACKINTOSH

Coffee has become a societal staple, but because of that, there is also widespread malpractice when it comes to making and consuming the beverage. Coffee flavors sell everything from chocolate to ice cream, and caffeine is used to make other types of food and drink more addictive so that more products will sell.

It is accurate, then, to say that coffee has pervaded society to the point where you need to take personal responsibility for the way that you use it because of the poor practices out there. In this chapter, I am going to take you through some hard lessons about coffee.

Hiding Caffeine: Commercial Abuse for Profit

Caffeine, as you now know, is a highly addictive drug. It is wonderful—do not get me wrong—but it has caused serious ripple effects in the world of commercial product sales. Companies have discovered that by adding caffeine to their food and drinks, they can sell a lot more products than if those same items were caffeine-free.

This troubling trend has become so widely adopted that the Food and Drug Administration was forced to open investigations into commercial brands adding caffeine to a growing number of products. Wrigley's, a popular gum manufacturer, has released a new type of gum that contains as much caffeine as a half a cup of coffee in each piece.

The FDA goes on to say that caffeine can be found in anything from jelly beans, oatmeal, waffles, syrup, gum, energy water, marshmallows, and energized sunflower seeds. There are consequences to this trend that are already being felt in society today.

Stress levels are off the charts, with 77%[20] of all U.S. citizens experiencing physical symptoms of stress on a regular basis. That is astounding! Even more astounding are the rates of disease associated with the inflammation that stress causes in the human body. Adding a stimulant like caffeine to food is having disastrous consequences in our society.

It is boosting disease and death rates, and it is actively contributing to the obesity epidemic. When your stress hormone, cortisol, is sky high, your body is told to create new fat cells—urgently. You gain weight when you overuse caffeine. This is why understanding the commercial threat is so important to this diet.

Regulating Personal Caffeine Levels: Coffee Crunch

Coffee is the most natural and the healthiest way to get your daily fixed dose of beneficial caffeine. But this means cutting out all other forms of caffeine in your life. In a world that demands constant energy and an "on-the-go" lifestyle, this will not be as easy as you think. The first step is calculating your personal caffeine score.

20   Stress Statistics, http://www.statisticbrain.com/stress-statistics/

Remember that any more than 400mg is considered "unsafe" by many medical establishments, but the ideal target is around 200–300 mg for a small dose. Just three cups of filter coffee, one energy drink, a chocolate, and a cup of tea will put you 300 mg over the limit.

In order to rein in your caffeine levels, you need to find out how much of it you consume in your normal day. Follow these rules, and record your data in a notebook.

- Check how much caffeine is in your daily cup of coffee. How many do you have on a normal day? Write down the amount.
- Look at all of your food inside your fridge and cupboard and record if there is any caffeine added to those products. When do you eat them? Write it down.
- Make a note to ask your favorite local coffee shop how much caffeine is in their average cup of coffee. Write it down!

The most likely culprits in your food cupboard are the packaged foods as opposed to the fresh ones. Get into the habit of reading food labels for your health. Aside from caffeine, food contains a lot of additives and extras that can make it harder to lose fat over time.

If you do not regulate your caffeine levels this way, you may not experience the same optimized fat loss that I did. Even worse, you may experience caffeine withdrawal or have significant caffeine cravings when you adjust your levels.

- It is important that you maintain low caffeine levels in your body so that it can properly metabolize food and break down fat.

Again, I would target low caffeine specialty coffee made from Arabica beans. Instant coffee is fine, but a lot of it has massive amounts of caffeine in it. There are 30 million people[21] in the U.S. right now drinking five or more cups of this coffee every day. Time

---

21   Caffeine Addiction Becomes a National Issue, http://www.caffeineawareness.org/
caffeineawarness4page.pdf

for a change! Think quality over quantity to really soak up all the benefits of the Café Diet.

Do a week-long test run of your new coffee habit to get your levels right. If you feel better on 150 mg of caffeine instead of 300 mg, then that is your ideal amount. Everyone is different, and that is important to remember. I had a friend who could consume high doses of caffeine and would still sleep soundly at night with no problems.

The Damaging Effects of Energy Drinks

The Journal of Pediatrics recently conducted a study that found out caffeine addiction is rising so rapidly that there has been a shift from soda drinking to energy drinks consumption. Energy drinks are well known carriers of various central nervous system stimulants—the most popular being caffeine of course.

Reasons that have been cited by these medical establishments are "health reasons" and "marketing," which is alarming to say the least. Because soda is now seen as an unhealthy food choice, there has been a rise in "energy-boosting" drinks because our Western society glorifies the ability to be focused and dynamic 24/7.

There are movements in the medical industry to curb the tide of energy drink adoption among kids and teens, but the truth is that no one who aims to be healthy and lose fat should consume these beverages.

They give you the false impression of helping you lose fat while they prevent you from doing so. In fact, to properly understand the urgent state of the energy drinks industry, let's have a look at a few types of drink and what their caffeine content is today.

- Your average can of Red Bull will contain 80 mg of caffeine, about the same as your average cup of instant coffee.

- It is a fact that Consumer Reports[22] has found that 11 energy drink labels do not even contain the amount of added caffeine anywhere on the product. You could be consuming 242 mg of caffeine at a time, and you would not know.

- Of the 16 other energy drink brands tested, 20% of them contained *more* caffeine than the label indicated. This is completely misguiding for someone that wants to maintain normal levels in their diet.

As a rule, you should limit your consumption of energy drinks. Most of them cause a spike in caffeine in your body, which leads to serious side effects. Some side effects include restlessness, insomnia, tremors, jittery speech, abnormal heart rhythms, and even seizures.

- Even though some of the best energy drinks contain less caffeine than your normal cup of coffee, they are often combined with alcohol, which is dangerous. Consuming four to five energy drinks in one evening can cause a severe caffeine overdose.

- Keep in mind that the moment you begin to experience the negative side effects of caffeine, you have reached your threshold.

If you are a big fan of energy drinks, think about reducing your intake or switching to something a little less caffeine-riddled. Going on this diet will only work if you maintain low caffeine levels in your body.

Soda and Caffeine Laden Sugar Highs

So which products in particular are causing issues because of their hidden caffeine content? I would have to say—aside from energy drinks—beer, soda, and candy. Interestingly, these products are targeted towards younger people, who need to work longer hours, stay up late, and work harder than they used to have to years ago.

---

22   Daniel DeNoon, How Much Caffeine Is in Your Energy Drink?, http://www.webmd.com/food-recipes/news/20121025/how-much-caffeine-energy-drink

Caffeine in beer has caused so much trouble that the Center for Science and Public Interest eventually sued MillerCoors to take their beverage, "Sparks," off the shelf.[23] It contained an astounding 214 mg of caffeine per can, and that is six times more than the average can of Coke.

While you are at it, take a closer look at all of your alcohol choices. Drinking caffeine, a nervous system stimulant, along with alcohol, a nervous system depressant, can cause havoc in your body anyway.

- Soda is a dangerous cocktail because it contains fairly high levels of caffeine and sugar, which is a lethal combo. The latest Gallup poll indicates that even though people know soda is bad for them, 48% of Americans[24] still drink it every day. If you want to control your caffeine intake, you have to cut out soda.

Caffeine-laden sugar highs are another huge problem in society today. Time after time, you will find caffeine added to all sorts of sugary candies and sweets. That means that you have the caffeine content and the sugar to deal with.

This is particularly destructive because caffeine can cause the human body to store all of that sugar as fat, which can end up as pre-diabetes, or a problem with insulin in your body. Candy[25] usually contains about 1–10 mg of caffeine, which adds up the more of it that you eat.

Not only do these foods cause mood disturbances, they cause "crashes" in your blood sugar levels that can result in dizziness and other awful side effects. If you have a sweet tooth and love to eat hard candy or sweets, take a look at the caffeine content beforehand.

23   Sarah, Klein, 12 Surprising Sources of Caffeine, http://magazine.foxnews.com/food-wellness/12-surprising-sources-caffeine

24   American Soda Consumption: Half of Us Drink It Everyday, Study Says, http://www.huffingtonpost.com/2012/07/25/half-of-americans-drink-soda-everyday-consumption_n_1699540.html

25   Caffeine in Food, http://www.caffeineinformer.com/caffeine-in-candy

- Cookies can contain 19 mg of caffeine.
- Marshmallows can contain 8 mg of caffeine.
- Soft candy can contain 6 mg or more of caffeine.
- Frozen yogurt contains 8 mg of caffeine or more.

If you have a "bad eating" day, you could be consuming as much as 200 mg of caffeine in sweets, soda, and cookies before you have even factored coffee into your life. It is important that you make note of this and insist on buying "treats" that are low in sugar or do not contain any sugar—and no caffeine.

The Ice Cream and Chocolate Debacle

Everyone loves the taste of creamy, yummy ice cream, but did you know that many ice creams are now packing an extra punch? These caffeine-based ice creams are hot sellers. And it is not just the chocolate varieties that are causing problems.

Caffeine can be present in syrups that are being used in the ice creams as well. That means that you should check the caffeine content of your ice cream before you eat it. Just one scoop of coffee or chocolate flavored ice cream can contain up to 80 mg of caffeine.

Better ice cream alternatives include vanilla or strawberry, but you will have to check if there is no caffeine infused in the sugary syrups that manufacturers are adding to make these treats more delicious and dopamine inducing.

Chocolate contains natural sources of caffeine from the cocoa bean, and these are usually in low levels and do not cause much trouble. Your average chocolate bar contains about 8 mg of caffeine, which is not much. The real trouble comes in again when you take a look at the combined sugar and caffeine effect.

Chocolate is an ingredient that has made its way into all sorts of different food choices. You can buy chocolate biscuits, cakes, rolls, milkshakes, alcohol, sweets, cereals, ice cream, yogurt, and even meat dipped in chocolate. If you love chocolate, you may want to think about switching to all natural 90% dark chocolate.

It contains the least amount of caffeine and sugar, and you can safely consume a few blocks of it along with your normal daily meals without worrying about health consequences. That said, now is the time to ransack your cupboard to forage for all the food items that contain chocolate. You can assume if it does, there is caffeine in there.

If you eat these daily, you may have to change to new brands or types of food to maintain your diet plan. Otherwise, factoring them into your daily caffeine count is all right. If on Tuesday you only want to consume two cups of coffee and have a scoop of dark chocolate ice cream, then that is fine as long as most other sugar sources are gone.

You can continue to eat chocolate in the form of cocoa with other sweeteners or natural sweet replacements. As always, it is best to train yourself to enjoy chocolate without sugar. It gives you all the health and endorphin benefits without any of the sugar damage.

- Understand that when you are eating ice cream or chocolate, there is a very good chance that you are consuming caffeine. Ask about it if you are at a restaurant.
- Make small changes to reduce the amount of caffeine that you consume so that you are guaranteed to lose fat when you begin your new nutrition plan.

Pain Killers, Energy Water, and Breakfast Caffeine

Caffeine is a marvelous substance when used in low doses. For that exact reason, it has been added to some not-so-conventional products for health benefits. The problem, of course, is that when an uneducated buyer consumes these products, they have no idea that they are contributing to their caffeine addiction and cortisol levels.

Medical research discovered that caffeine in low doses has a mild painkiller effect, and it can even ease muscle pain. Interestingly, researchers also found that it improves the effectiveness of over-the-counter pain medication, although they are not sure why.

Painkillers, therefore, contain caffeine. Some painkillers contain small doses of caffeine, and others contain as much as your average cup of coffee. Either way, they are still contributing to your caffeine intake. Take certain types of extra strength aspirin for example— they contain 65 mg of caffeine.

If you have a headache and you decide to take aspirin, you need to factor that in. Just two pills can have you at the tipping point if you drink the same amount of coffee that day. Then there are other hidden caffeine sources, like energy water.

Energy water can range from different types of vitamin water with added caffeine to various types of flavored water with added caffeine. This product exemplifies society's fascination with caffeine. It is basically selling drinkable caffeine with little else.

Many of these waters contain about 80–90 mg of caffeine in them—about as much as a cup of morning coffee. But there are variants that climb as high as 200 mg per bottle. These are dangerous enough and should not be used lightly, or at all, if you love coffee.

Finally, and perhaps the most disturbing of all the caffeine laced products, is the new trend of adding caffeine to breakfast cereals. That means eating caffeine while drinking caffeine in the morning— it is just too much.

Everything from oatmeal to chocolate bran flakes are being infused with added caffeine so that supermarkets can sell more boxes of the stuff. Do not even get me started on the brands that use chocolate then add even more caffeine and skew the content on the box.

There are bad practices everywhere, and I would encourage you to avoid cereals altogether. They are usually full of sugar and have almost no real nutritional value anyway. You are better off eating fruit, eggs, and other real food sources that are naturally caffeine free.

To recap, you need to avoid accidentally supplementing your diet with caffeine when you eat at home or when you go out to eat. It is important that you focus on maintaining your caffeine levels while you are eating according to the Café Diet rules.

I promise that if you can maintain the right caffeine levels, this diet will help you quickly and effectively shed those extra pounds before your next big event. These are short-term fat loss tips, but they can really be applied every day if you can manage it.

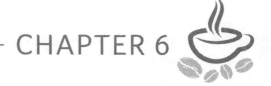

CHAPTER 6

Regulating Coffee for Sustained Fat Loss

"I like cappuccino, actually. But even a bad cup of coffee is better than no coffee at all."

DAVID LYNCH

Once you understand the ins and outs of coffee and its place in the world, the next step is to get cracking on your fat loss plan. It is true that I used these short burst diets to shed pounds and improve my overall health.

I did it with almost no exercise outside of my normal job, just a careful diet facilitated with the help of my favorite beverage, coffee. I have reduced my risk of contracting diabetes along with a host of life-threatening diseases that manifest along with it.

This chapter is about teaching you how to build and regulate a system for sustained weight loss using the correct food, the right coffee, and a positive mindset.

Putting Together Your Coffee Health Plan

When I was putting together my own coffee health plan, I focused on a few things to make the process easier and the journey speedy and efficient. Now, I am no dietician, doctor, or life coach. I have a college degree from an entirely different field of study. My goal for this fat loss diet was simple—lose fat fast with as little exercise as possible.

My job as a roast master is very demanding, so I had almost no extra time for the gym or any strenuous exercise. I think most people looking for a way to lose fat do not have time for huge exercise routines or long gym expeditions.

My social and family life deserved to get whatever remained after my busy work schedule, and I was not interested in sacrificing hours a day for a diet. Most of the day I am behind two ovens—my coffee roasters. You have to have a lot of energy and stamina for that, so I needed a diet that gave me enough energy and calories to do my job without passing out.

I experimented with many techniques and discovered some that worked well. The basis for the Café Diet comes from these principles.

- The diet has to be easy for a busy lifestyle.
- It has to be safe and healthy.
- It does not require social or exercise sacrifices.
- It does not involve mass food preparation.
- It includes trouble-free, intermittent fasting.
- It gives you enough calories for work.
- It provides a solution for overcoming perpetual hunger.

I will never forget fasting for the first time, quite by accident, and then realizing that I could use coffee to prevent the hunger pains that followed. I dug into a cup of Ethiopian Yirgacheffe and sipped on that until my hunger was gone.

You need to put your Café Diet plan together based on your own lifestyle. I am going to show you how by taking you through what worked best for me on my journey.

Setting Fat Loss Goals: SMART Caffeine

The first step of this fat loss plan is to consider your caffeine levels, which I have spoken about at some length. By now, your cupboards should contain only the caffeine sources you are aware of; everything else should be binned. You should also have reconsidered your involvement with fast food, processed food, and sugar by now.

This is because caffeine in high doses does not go well with these food types. They will prevent you from losing weight at every turn and will make fat loss impossible. The best thing to do is to start from scratch with a detox. Follow these SMART caffeine rules.

- Set **specific** caffeine goals for yourself. If you crave 600 mg of coffee, outline a schedule that takes you back down to 300 mg so that the diet can work. If your caffeine goals are not reached, you may struggle to stay hunger free.
- Set **measurable** caffeine goals for yourself. Quite literally, spend a small amount of time writing down on a chart, or in an app, the amount of caffeine you consume each time during the day while on your diet. Review and tweak your numbers. For healthy adults with no medical issues, it is generally agreed upon that 300 mg–400 mg of caffeine can be consumed daily without any adverse effects.[26]
- Set **attainable** caffeine goals for yourself. Caffeine is still a drug, and you need to know your body. If you are used to consuming high volumes of caffeine, or you are more of a decaf drinker (which still contains low dose caffeine), you need to be able to achieve your caffeine goals inside your lifestyle limitations.
- Set **realistic** caffeine goals for yourself. If you are an IT technician and you work very late nights, caffeine may be your

26 Caffeine Safe Limits: How to Determine Your Safe Daily Dose, http://www.caffeineinformer.com/caffeine-safe-limits

only driver. You will have to sit down and carefully examine your schedule, tolerance, and mindset to establish goals that are realistic.

- Set **timely** caffeine goals for yourself. The Café Diet can be limited to a certain amount of days, weeks, or months, or it can be more long term. But you ultimately decide, according to when you can consume your coffee and how easily this diet integrates into your life.

Once you have set your caffeine goals (not recommended to be more than 300-400mg) to combat hunger pangs, I suggest working out all of the other more technical details about your diet. This means knowing how much you weigh, what you have to lose, and what a SMART fat loss goal in that restricted time space looks like. Fat loss can be rapid, but work needs to be put in to keep the fat off.

I find that the larger you are, the quicker the fat melts off you with this diet. If, like me, you were under 30 pounds overweight, the process may be slower. Fast weight loss is not recommended by physicians anyway; it depends on your ability to maintain your caffeine levels, your nutritional choices, and your fasting regimen.

This diet is perfect for shedding a few instant pounds before an important event or occasion in your life. It is also great for figuring out how your body operates and responds to food as well as how you can use this to your advantage for healthy eating in your life.

Benchmarking Your Current Bad Habits

Step 2 is to figure out all of your essential metrics so that you can benchmark your current bad habits. One of the first things I did was figure out my ideal BMI. BMI stands for body mass index, and you can figure yours out using both the old and new methods. For tools and more information about the diet, please look at my website, www.thecafediet.com.

I am 172 cm tall, and my weight was 181 lb. I had an unhealthy BMI score of 27.5. Based on my age and activity level and my daily Basal Metabolic Rate, I needed to consume 2400 calories a day to stay at that weight.

I aimed for a BMI of 23.5. My "ideal" weight adjusted to 154 pounds, which was my new target. So I calculated my Basal Metabolic Rate according to my target weight. My new BMR was 2200 calories a day. I had to create a 200 calorie deficit every day to lose fat.

To accelerate this process, I reduced my calorie intake to 1800 calories a day, meaning that I created a 600 calorie shortage in my body. This made it possible to lose one pound every six days. Losing one pound a week is considered healthy fat loss, and it will stay off if monitored.

- Work out your current BMI according to old and new methods.
- Establish your BMR, and record the numbers.
- Work out what you want your BMI to be.
- Target your ideal BMR to achieve your fat loss goal.

For a week before I began my diet, I spent time benchmarking all of my old eating habits and poor practices. When I reviewed them, I realized that I had a lot of habits to change and work to do if the Café Diet was going to work for me.

You will have to do the same thing if you want to minimize your chances of derailing your diet. Simply grab a notebook and record your eating, sleeping, exercise, and daily routine habits. Then at the end of the week, review how you engage with food and how you can improve small things to result in your target BMR.

Benchmarking your current bad habits is excellent if you are one of the "eat on the go" types. Lots of people are not aware of how many calories they consume a day. You would be surprised. Only when you see a weeks' worth of your bad eating will you realize how far you have strayed off the path of health and wellness.

- Use applications on your smartphone to track and measure your progress. There are dozens of great free fat loss trackers out there. You can track your calories easily with the right app.
- Moderate calorie restriction works best in short bursts. If you want to lose three pounds, set up a three-week long Café Diet plan. Follow the diet, and you will lose three or more pounds by your target date.

Short- and Long-Term Fat Loss With Coffee

The Café Diet aims to never allow you to dip below 1800 calories because any less and your body might slip into starvation mode. When your body thinks that you are starving, it automatically begins to horde your calories.

As far as your body is concerned, you could be on a desert island and in dire need of conserved energy. Everything slows down, including fat loss. If you dip below the 1800-calorie mark, your body will turn to your muscles for calories and burn them.

The good news is that you can use the Café Diet for short- and long-term fat loss. The interesting thing is that you do not have to be on this diet all the time. You only need to eat fairly healthily on your off days or weeks.

- Short-term fat loss with coffee involves setting a timeline to lose one pound every six days in a healthy manner. The coffee will fend off the hunger pains, and it will facilitate your fasting process. More on that later.
- Long-term fat loss with coffee happens when you plan to use the Café Diet once a month or one month on, one month off—however you would like to structure it around your busy schedule.

For example, if you have to attend a family reunion in two months' time, you can engage the Café Diet to shed those five awkward pounds that are making you look frumpy. This is goal-orientated, short-term fat loss.

Simply outline your time schedule, and select the weeks that you want to stick to your Café Diet plan. Two months gives you eight weeks to choose from, so you can diet for five of them and eat normally for the other three.

A longer-term goal can involve any timeline, and it can be as gradual as you like. If you know you have to attend a special function like a wedding at the end of the year, add one week of the Café Diet to your month, every month. By the end of the year, you should have lost around 12 pounds—while eating normally most of the time.

I would encourage you to try to keep your coffee intake at Café Diet levels as often as possible. This is because your body will want to continue losing fat after each week, and if your cortisol levels jump, you may find that you gain back the pound you lost.

If this happens, find out why. Did you eat a lot of junk food or sugar? Did you drink a ton of coffee when you know how much caffeine you have put inside your body? Small factors like this matter, but they only take minutes of your day and self-control.

This is perfectly implementable for a busy person that wants to shed fat without any outrageous exercise programs going on.

Fast Coffee Fat Loss: Lose Pounds in Days

So how does the Café Diet use intermittent fasting to accelerate your fat loss and help you shed one solid pound every six days? The idea of intermittent fasting came to me through a friend who used it to control his weight issues.

Do you know why you eat three meals a day? Children may need to do this because they are growing, but adults are already fully grown. A hundred years ago people did not consume food three times a day, especially with "modern" high-calorie food; it is a modern convention. In fact, they ate when they were hungry.

In the U.S. alone, 70 million people are affected by digestive diseases.[27] We consume things our bodies cannot metabolize all the time. Fasting, on the other hand, gives your digestive system a much needed break from the barrage of foreign substances.

It was Hippocrates who said, "Death begins in the colon," which means that what we eat affects how we feel. Some 70% of the cells in your body's immune system[28] are found in the walls of your gut. That means what you eat affects how your body fights off illness.

In the Café Diet, intermittent fasting is the decision to skip certain meals during your diet. That means that you need to regularly eat at a specific time, preferably breakfast time, and then you can skip a lunch and eat a healthy, regular dinner. You can also choose to skip both lunch and dinner. The most important thing that you need to remember is to keep at least 10 hour breaks between meals. I usually eat a good breakfast around 7 a.m. and have dinner around 6 p.m. I do not recommend eating after 6 p.m., but it depends on your schedule. If you follow these rules, you have two "fasting" periods in a 24-hour day. One, approximately 10-11 hours between breakfast and dinner, and the other 10-11 hours in the night and before breakfast in the morning.

The most critical thing is to try to avoid any type of sugar during the fasting period. This is how you gain back your insulin sensitivity and detox your body. During that time, if you absolutely need it, just add a hint of half and half in your coffee. Even fat-free milk has enough sugar to ruin your effort. Half and half is sugar free.

When your body is in a state of fasting, it has no energy to burn, so it pulls fat stored in your body and burns that. This improves insulin sensitivity levels and stabilizes blood sugar. For fast coffee fat loss, your average day can look like this.

27   Digestive Diseases Statistics for the United States, http://digestive.niddk.nih.gov/statistics/statistics.aspx

28   Furness, JB, Kunze, WA, Nutrient Tasting and Signalling Mechanisms in The Gut, The Intestine As a Sensory Organ: Neural, Endocrine, and Immune Responses, http://www.ncbi.nlm.nih.gov/pubmed/10564096

- Have a large breakfast as the main meal of the day. Have a good dinner but skip lunch. A fasting state happens for 10–12 hours depending on your choice.

Fasting not only helps you lose fat, it increases growth hormone production in your body. This means that insulin sensitivity will rise and your body will be primed for muscle growth, which facilitates any natural exercise that you get during the day.

- The Café Diet works in six-day cycles. One pound should come off your body every six days. During your six-day cycle, you should use intermittent fasting as a way of accelerating your fat loss.

Everyone is different remember? Sometimes people will love the idea of intermittent fasting and will take to it immediately. Others will struggle. The key is to continue to use coffee when you feel the pull of hunger. As long as you keep your caffeine levels low, you can put an end to any persuasive hunger pains.

Sustained Coffee Fat Loss: Lose Pounds Over Months

For sustained fat loss, this plan works along with any busy schedule. Like I mentioned earlier, fasting can cause hunger issues. When I started my first Café Diet cycle, by lunchtime—after I had skipped the lunch part—I was very hungry.

A lot of diet books tell you to drink water to eliminate hunger, but too much water just made me feel sick and even hungrier. To get the water in—and the caffeine—coffee was the best choice. A hot cup of Arabica with no sugar was all I needed to chase away those extreme hunger pains. Just drink a cup of coffee and on you get with your work.

To understand why caffeine takes away hunger, you need to understand how leptin works in your body. Leptin[29] was discovered in 1995 and has since been of great interest to scientists seeking new treatments for Type 2 diabetes and obesity. Leptin, like insulin, is a hormone. It is part of a network of regulatory hormones that control how energy is consumed and used up in the body. Resistance to leptin, or a lack of it, has been associated with obesity. Leptin is also a protein that your fat cells manufacture. It circulates in your blood and works on your brain. Leptin will tell your brain if your fat cells contain enough energy for normal bodily function. If not, a hunger alarm is raised.

When you lose fat, the amount of leptin that you produce decreases. That means with every pound that you lose, you will be less hungry over time. But it also means that your body will think that the lack of leptin means that you are starving. Hunger pains result.

The Gallae warriors of Ethiopia used to carry around caffeine-rich fat balls of crushed coffee to ward off hunger on long military expeditions. Since then, coffee has been used by numerous people to abate hunger. It is even added to weight loss pills and supplements for this reason. To control your fasting, you need to drink coffee!

- Sustained coffee fat loss will involve the use of coffee to reduce your hunger pains while you are in the midst of a Café Diet cycle. Every cycle is six days long, and with another six to eight hours of fasting on that, you will need at least two cups of coffee to deal with the hunger pangs later in the day.

- People often sip on coffee throughout the day when they are on these cycles. You do not have to drink an entire cup of coffee all at once. Caffeine takes a while to kick in, and it stays and compounds in your body during the day. Slow release of it in low doses means you will be hunger free all day.

29 Overcoming Leptin Resistance in the Battle Against Obesity, http://www.medicalnewstoday.com/articles/251429.php

Using these simple principles, you can use the Café Diet to lose pounds over a period of several months. No one can be expected to diet and lose weight all of the time. Instead, by adding these fat loss cycles to your month, you can lose fat over time and enjoy some of the more decadent foods that you are not allowed to eat on a diet.

Of course, I am not referring to anything with sugar in it or processed food. These are just destructive food products that cause ill health and harm in your body. When you consume them regularly, your chances of losing fat rapidly decline.

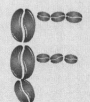

Is for Food: Pairing Coffee With Nutrition

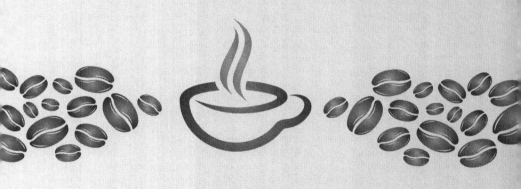

CHAPTER 7

The Skinny on Healthy Food Choices: Brunch

I am a coffee fanatic. Once you go to proper coffee, you can't go back. You cannot go back."
HUGH LAURIE

Now that you know how to structure and implement your diet, I am going to take a closer look at the various types of food choices that go well with the Café Diet. These choices are just as important as the coffee itself, and they work hand in hand for fat loss.

In section III, you will learn how to make the right nutrition choices now that you are fully aware of the foods to cut out of your diet. Follow these very simple rules, and like me, you will find your body reshaping itself as the months sweep by.

Your Breakfast Food Pairing Chart

Breakfast is the most important meal of the day. In the Café Diet, it should be one of your main meals of the day, so it has to be very impressive and nutrient rich. Keeping in mind that you should not be consuming cereals or other high sugar breakfast choices, here is how you should go about pairing coffee with your breakfast.

- Gorgeous Costa Rican coffee, medium roast, pairs well with a classic egg breakfast. Scramble, fry, poach, or boil your eggs, and eat along with tomato, high quality non-processed sausage, a salad, and two slices of wheat-free bread.

- If you like to bake, prepare an egg, spinach, tomato, and mushroom quiche for breakfast—and have a sizable portion. Quiches and similar egg-based bakes pair well with French roasts and Pacific Island blends.

- Egg salad can also be a satisfying breakfast if you add in carbohydrate-based vegetables like butternut, beetroot, or other richer veggies. Experiment with different egg salad combos, and enjoy two eggs in your salad. Pair these with the richer, nuttier dark roast coffees for a flavor boost.

A single egg is one of the most nutritious forms of food in the world. In recent years it has been discovered that the once "evil" chicken egg does not, in fact, cause cholesterol issues. For 40 years the medical establishment swore that eggs were the cause of high blood pressure, high cholesterol, and increased risk for heart attacks and other concerns.

The truth is that fifty years ago when people were eating tons of eggs—and little sugar—they were in better health. Eggs contain excellent nutrients that your body needs to keep going and remain in peak condition. Recent studies[30] have found that there is absolutely no connection between eating eggs daily and increased rates of heart disease.

Breakfast foods will need to become more creative if you are going to skip dinner. Packing them with nutrients and not carbohydrates is

---

30   Katherine, Tallmadge, Eggs Don't Deserve Their Bad Reputation Studies Show (Op-Ed), http://www.livescience.com/39353-eggs-dont-deserve-bad-reputation.html

a tough thing to do. Try to avoid eating too much bread or anything that contains too much sugar.

The Coffee and Fruit Revelation

If you desperately miss the sugar in your coffee, there are ways to drink coffee that make it sweeter and more enjoyable. I am a huge advocate of getting your sugar intake from fruit over any other source. Fruit is often high in natural sugars, so you should target the lower end of the spectrum—strawberries, plums, watermelon, and other stone fruits.

To pair your sweet fruit with coffee, you will need to find out which flavors match and how they will present themselves with your chosen fruit or fruit combo. Eating these together is an absolute revelation because you get all that sweetness from the fruit with the delicate flavor of your coffee choices. Here is how to pair them.

- Dark or medium roast Brazilian coffees and Costa Rican blends work very well with baked fruit. If you decide to create a simple, low-sugar fruit tart, you can match these blends with your food for an additional flavor burst.

- Haitian coffee and Tanzanian coffee are very distinct and pair well with any number of simple stone fruits. In fact, I found that after a while I did not want to enjoy fruits like plums without some unique coffee to go along with it.

- Jamaican and Yemeni coffees are fresh and interesting, and they taste great when you pair them with berries. Strawberries, gooseberries, loganberries, blueberries—get your hands on a mix of these super fruits, and add some to your daily breakfast regimen for the nutritional content.

- Latin American coffees are known for their intense, tangy flavors, and these will pair well with any number of citrus fruits. Keep in mind that fruit alone is not enough for your breakfast. Focus on multiple sources of nutrition, and combine them into a power-packed meal.

- Arabian and African coffees are spicy and have notes of cocoa in them. You can pair these types of coffee with fruit that is naturally sweet—like your citrus varieties. The more enjoyment that you get from your coffee, the better your diet will go.

If you need to get in some muesli or something similar, dial down the carb-heavy muesli and add more fruit to the bowl. Reversing the bulk of the bowl is a trick that adds sweetness to your breakfast, minimizes carb intake, and contributes to your daily fiber needs.

As a side note, coffee from Guatemala is especially good with a fruit like apples because it sets off those bittersweet notes. At the end of the day, you need to see what appeals to your palate the most. I have gone on other people's recommendations with coffee only to discover that I found great pleasure in matching my own coffee to food.

In the Café Diet, you should be eating a few fruit items every day to get the nutrients that you need for health and wellness. You also need fuel to burn, which means that every nutrient matters. With fruit, there is more nutritional value because it is mainly eaten raw.

Enjoying Coffee and Chocolate for Fat Loss

A good brunch is not complete without some kind of chocolate in there. The average person may eat candy every day or chocolate a few times a week. The truth is that it is not the chocolate that is bad for you but the sugar that they put in your chocolate.

The obvious solution then becomes finding a type of chocolate that is low in sugar and pairs well with coffee. This type of chocolate requires a period of enjoyment, contemplation, and calm when you are eating it with coffee.

Replacing your old chocolate and candy habits this way is very helpful. Simply cut out all other forms of chocolate and only buy

90% dark chocolate or an equivalent. Dark chocolate contains concentrated forms of cocoa and some caffeine, so check on that.

The dark chocolate is actually beneficial for your health as long as you restrict yourself to a maximum of two to three blocks per day. Focus on pairing a blend of coffee that can compete with the cocoa notes in your dark chocolate.

- A cup of instant or filter coffee, brewed black, or a shot of espresso pair well with two normal blocks of very dark chocolate. The chocolate is meant to be eaten on the side of the coffee plate as an alternative to sugar.
- A dark hazelnut chocolate should be paired with a rich, full-bodied coffee. There are different methods of eating the chocolate with the coffee to enhance the flavor and enjoyment of the process.

To properly enjoy your dark chocolate and coffee experience, follow these eating methods. First you will need to admire and appreciate the aroma of the coffee and how it mingles with and complements the aroma of the dark chocolate.

During your first small bite of the chocolate you should take note of how the chocolate snaps because that indicates quality and texture. From this point, you have a lot of options. Sometimes it tastes great to hold the dark chocolate in your mouth and let it melt against the roof there. Other times dipping your chocolate in your coffee is fun and delicious.

Dark chocolate gives you that intense cocoa fix that you crave. Often it is the cocoa that you want and not the sugar, yet normal chocolate is mainly sugar, so you cannot get it from there. Try Asian and specifically Indonesian coffees for their low acid content and bold flavors.

You can also try Arabia and African coffees; they are medium-range acidity, but their distinct floral aromas work particularly well with chocolate. I would suggest always keeping a slab of dark chocolate in your fridge in case you feel like something nice.

But it is important that you slow down and take the time to enjoy eating your chocolate. You want to experience the flavor instead of wolfing down the sugar.

The Rich Omelet: Stuffed With Goodness

One of the best types of breakfast food is the omelet. This is because it gives you the egg content that you need while enabling you to fill the middle with other nutrients. And there is literally no limit on how much nutrition you can cram into your omelet.

You would not know it to look at it, but there are dozens of ways to prepare an omelet—and with the unlimited fillings, you can prepare yourself a breakfast that will take care of all of your nutritional needs in one sitting.

- There are microwavable omelets for when you are feeling lazy, omelets made in bags, German omelets, and 40-second omelets. You can cook them on the stove, in the oven, or in a frying pan.
- Omelets go well with a meat choice like bacon and accompanying ingredients. These can be anything from feta, mushrooms, peppers, spinach, and kale to jalapenos, onions, tomatoes, and broccoli. It depends on what you like, but I would encourage you to go big.
- Traditionally, Indonesian and Sumatran Java coffee roasts are excellent for savory omelets. But I would not limit myself here. A dash of milk in any of these blends can round off the taste so that they pair well.

Enjoy different omelet styles and cooking methods, and add various protein sources like sausage, bacon, mince, and chicken to give your dish more nutrient power. Cheese usually pairs well with black coffee only, so be careful of adding tons of oily cheese to your brunch.

I was never into omelets until I realized that they were like a healthier way of eating an egg-based burrito without any negative side effects at all. Now I actively look for things to stuff my omelets with because they are such a great breakfast and an ongoing source of energy for me during the day.

Something else to look at if you like, are seafood omelets. They require more prep time and are quite difficult to get right. That said, they contain a lot of great nutrients for you, so if you are a seafood lover, eat seafood omelets!

A rich omelet prepares you for your day and takes away that lasting hunger. Many scientists have called it "nature's natural appetite suppressant" because it keeps the human body fuller for longer. In a study conducted by U.S. researchers,[31] eggs were found to suppress appetite a lot more effectively than cereals.

If, like me, you constantly find yourself starving by 11 a.m., eating eggs each day will help you control that. Pair it with coffee, which also has an appetite suppressing mechanism, and you should be able to last quite comfortably until the next day or later that evening.

Sweet, Savory, and Light Breakfast Pairings

Coffee is a champion of breakfast meals. In fact, I would bet that you are drinking coffee along with your normal breakfast every day. But everyone is different. I will not assume to understand your cultural differences or how they affect your eating habits.

What I can do is give you a more solid idea on how to pair coffee with your breakfast because it is going to become such a staple in

---

31   Fiona, Macrae, Why Eggs for Breakfast Will Keep Those Hunger Pangs Away Until Lunchtime, http://www.dailymail.co.uk/health/article-2143181/Why-eggs-breakfast-hunger-pangs-away-lunchtime.html

your life. When you match the right food with coffee, it not only makes the food taste better, it makes the coffee taste better too.

- Sumatran coffee matches well with mushrooms, beef, and flavors that are more woody and earthy. These are savory flavors.
- Ethiopian coffee is excellent with chicken, lemon flavors, and lime. It goes the best with lighter flavors.
- Jamaican coffee is great with blueberries and other sweet fruits.
- Costa Rican coffee is wonderful with some baked goods as long as they are light and contain fruit.
- Java is the best choice for soft cheeses, fresh herbs, and mushrooms for those tangy notes in savory dishes.
- Brazilian, Mexican, Hawaiian, and Yemeni coffees pair superbly with sweet things, especially chocolate and types of fruit.

When you build your breakfast or brunch, keep in mind that there may be ingredients here that contain caffeine. Check everything as you assemble the recipe. Keep notes on how your breakfast tastes and if the coffee matches well with the food according to your palate.

I once went to an upmarket restaurant and was served a coffee and omelet pairing that was hideous. The coffee was ultra-bitter and the spinach in the omelet was equally as bitter. The result was a very bitter affair indeed and one I would not repeat.

For sweet flavors, you want to go for the more complex coffee flavors found in your robust Arabica beans. A nice spicy blend will also go well on occasion with chocolate and fruit. The lighter flavors are harder to pair, but you can choose a medium range coffee that tastes great and still complements the delicate flavors of your breakfast.

Savory is the easiest to pair because you can play around with those rich, nutty, creamy, and intense flavors that can overpower other types of food. There is nothing more satisfying than sipping on an intense cup of coffee while enjoying a rich, savory omelet.

I noticed that the longer I was on the Café Diet, the more time I took to enjoy my food. Instead of just gobbling it down like I used to do, I could enjoy the flavors and the pairing, and I took my time with each bite. This made eating a whole new experience for me.

Navigating Breakfast Restaurant Foods: Coffee Please

You are not going to eat at home for the rest of your life, so let's talk about eating out at restaurants. There are some things that you need to watch out for and others that you should completely steer clear of in various restaurant scenarios.

- Most menus only contain a few different types of coffee. Figure out how they can best serve it to you by selecting your style. Avoid the sugar on the foam decoration.

- The average restaurant cooks with sunflower or canola oil, which is not very healthy for you at all. You should focus on cooking with olive oil or butter only. When you cut sugar out of your diet, you can eat butter with no adverse side effects. Always ask if you can pay extra to have your food cooked with olive oil.

- Look in your area to see if there are any coffee and food pairing restaurants out there. The trend is gaining ground, and more of these restaurants are supporting the idea that coffee pairing can be just as complex as wine pairing.

- Try to go to restaurants where they serve organic food or at least give you an option to choose healthier dishes. Avoid fast food chains and big brand restaurants because these are the places where you will gain weight—even if you order a "healthier" option.

- Do not eat the bread that they offer you with every egg dish on the menu. This bread contains more sugar and ill health than anything else on your plate. If you are going to order a salad, then ask your waiter to keep the salad dressing off the salad. Those dressings contain loads of sugar, and they turn a good meal into a bad one.

There is a good reason why you focus on egg dishes for breakfast in the Café Diet. This is because if you try to order a protein and vegetable dish for breakfast, it may not contain enough nutrients, and you will get hungry before your fast begins.

That said, if you crave some red meat, add it to an omelet. Be willing to stick to this plan to see how it goes. Within a week or two the differences will be astounding. You have no idea how much rubbish you are putting in your system until you cut it out.

For now, the rule is if you do not know, ask. You are allowed to be picky in a world where restaurant owners make decisions on free range or battery, hormones or clean food. Always demand free range, organic, natural sources of food to stay healthy.

CHAPTER 8

The Skinny on Healthy Food Choices: Dinner

"No one can understand the truth until he drinks of coffee's frothy goodness."
SHEIK ABD-AL-KABIR

If you decide to use intermittent fasting at lunch or in the morning, you will need a food pairing chart so that you can select healthy dinner choices. If you prefer to eat a large dinner and skip brunch, then you can do it this way as well.

The fat loss may be slower, but it will work because of the careful calorie intake. You need to get the skinny on healthy dinner choices and how coffee can enhance them. In this chapter, you will find out how to do that and how fasting will work for your body.

Your Dinner Food Pairing Chart

Eating large dinners in the evening is not recommended, but let's face it, there will be times when you have to eat out or eat dinner at night. Nothing in life is ever really fixed. To prepare you for this, you need to know how to pair dinner foods with coffee.

The same principles exist for the breakfast section, although the complexity of flavors is really up to the individual. One of my favorite is a starit French roast Costa Rica. It is very unique and earthy, and it is incredible with cheeses. Yet traditionally, these blends are not meant to be paired with cheese.

- As a rule, sweet foods for dinner need coffees from Jamaica, Brazil, and Mexico because they complement the lingering sweetness that you like as you drink your coffee. So not only is your coffee slightly sweeter, your food tastes more complex because of the notes in your coffee.

- Savory foods need a richer, darker, and more intense type of coffee bean. I would suggest pairing these Sumatran blends with roasts and a side of vegetables or salad. The meal is healthy, is widely available at restaurants, and will not affect your fat loss plan.

- Light foods like salads and other delicate dinner options need to go with your lighter roasted coffee blends and your grocery store instant coffees. A creamier coffee is great with a crisp salad, but if you are going for a vegetable dish, you may want to get something a little more intense to balance out the flavors.

Dinnertime is not the best time to eat a large and heavy meal, especially not on the rush, quick mode. You have spent the whole day working, and now you have a million and five things to do. But first you have to eat something because you will be sick if you do not. That is what the average American's dinner time has become. Every day when I am driving home from work, I am surprised how long the lines are waiting in the fast food drive thru.

To avoid this, I strongly suggest fasting through dinner at least some of the time on the Café Diet. See how it goes. It can be invigorating eating a huge meal at breakfast and a small snack at supper time.

How Coffee Can Accompany Dinner Foods

Traditionally, it is not uncommon to find unique rules in European countries about when and how to drink coffee with your dinner. In Italy, they have an unspoken rule about cappuccino that has resulted in many glaring looks if you sit in an Italian bistro after 11 a.m. with one.

Italians believe that the milk in your coffee corrupts the digestive system, so they feel the best time to drink cappuccino is before breakfast or with breakfast. But the concept is interesting if you want to try to use coffee as a digestive at dinnertime. Cut out the milk!

- If you are going to drink coffee with your dinner, make sure it is an early dinner at about 5 p.m. in the evening. Caffeine will stay in your system for a very long time after that, which may reduce the quality of the sleep that you get that night.

- Test a few days with milk and a few days without milk to see if your digestive system has any changes. I know some people that swear blind about this milk thing, so it is definitely worth trying out for your physiology.

- In Western society, it is normal to drink coffee after dinner. In fact, it is normal to drink coffee all the time. Walk into any diner or restaurant and there is every chance that a coffee pot touting waitress will offer you some. When you are in these types of situations, avoid drinking coffee after lunchtime if you can, and aim to have it before, not after, your meal.

- If you are like the French, you drink coffee all day, every day. That does not mean they overdo their caffeine; it just means that their choices are different. Most French drink their coffee with dinner—and they have it in espresso form with no milk.

- The French are coffee snobs; they do not drink many coffee blends. Instead, they swear by individual flavors. By putting flavor ahead of caffeine, they can consume more coffee, even at dinnertime. Plus, by pouring boiling water over fresh beans, some of the caffeine is destroyed by the heat. Your average French espresso has less caffeine in it than a normal cup of American instant.

You need to decide how you are going to enjoy coffee with your various dinner foods. That means being a guinea pig like me for a bit. I strongly encourage you to have a week-long test run of fasting on breakfast and then switch to fasting on dinner to see which works best for your lifestyle. Most of the time, breakfast always wins.

Aim for Arabica-based coffees to keep the caffeine content low. You can even choose to drink decaf if you are out at night and want a little caffeine. The University of Florida[32] did a study on decaffeinated coffee and discovered that the process does not rid the coffee of caffeine—it merely reduces the amount.

You can cheat the caffeine fix by drinking decaf in the evenings so that you can still benefit from the other elements in coffee. About 10 cups of decaf is the equivalent of two to three cups of normal coffee. If you love coffee but are sensitive to caffeine, switch to decaf with your evening meals.

Limiting Grains and Carbs: The Sugar Trap

If you are groaning about my recommendation to steer clear of dinner, this is probably because your dinner is very carbohydrate rich and acts on your brain to create the illusion of happiness, enjoyment, and satiety at the end of your day.

I have already spoken to you about sugar, but worse than raw sugar are the dozens of carbohydrates that hide sugar. When you eat a carb, it becomes sugar in your body, so it is really the exact same thing as eating sugar; it just takes a little longer to metabolize.

---

32 Decaffeinated Coffee Is Not Caffeine-Free, Experts Say, http://www.sciencedaily.com/releases/2006/10/061012185602.htm

Limiting grains and high carbohydrate foods should become a lifestyle choice for you if you want to keep your fat off. This is because carbs were designed to help you gain fat. How these grains made it onto the government's recommended healthy eating pyramid is beyond me; they have skewed the food scale and destroyed a lot of healthy bodies.

You cannot walk into a supermarket anymore without having a thousand grain-based products thrown at you. Grain products sell fast, and people always come back for more. Grain, in other words, is big, big business. But it is also very unhealthy for your body—especially a body that wants to shed some pounds.

The bottom line is that the human digestive system has not evolved to digest grains properly. They were originally grown to be a quick source of energy. They were never meant to take over the entire Western diet. Most grains and high carbohydrates are vicious sugar traps that will spike your blood sugar and cause serious inflammation in your body.

According to the latest research by Dr. David Perlmutter,[33] when you eat too many grains and carbs, it dulls your brain, which can lead to all sorts of neurological disorders later in life. Grain keeps your body "high" on sugar, which causes inflammation—the starting point for all of today's modern diseases. He blames our high carb diets for our high disease rates.

I am not sure if this is 100% true or not, but what I do know is what has worked for me. I limit my grains and dense carbs and experience exceptional health benefits because of it. Did my mental performance seem to improve a few weeks later? Yes it did. But I have no idea if your physiology will be the same; you have to test it first.

---

33   Max, Lugavere, Your Healthy Diet Could Be Quietly Killing Your Brain, http://www.psychologytoday.com/blog/the-optimalist/201310/your-healthy-diet-could-be-quietly-killing-your-brain

My advice for the Café Diet is to limit your intake of grains, processed flours, and carbohydrates. If you can, segment your meals so that only 10% of them contain carbs of some form. Carbohydrates include heavily starchy vegetables like potatoes and grains like bread, pasta, and other baked goods.

If you have to eat a carbohydrate, I suggest eating rice. At least there are nutrients in it that your body can use, and it has not gone through any chemical processes. Just cutting out most of your grains and carbs alone should help the caffeine in your coffee do its work.

If you have too many carbs, no amount of coffee will stave off your hunger. It is a precarious balance, but it must be struck for good health and wellness.

The Secret of Intermittent Fasting

I spoke briefly about intermittent fasting earlier on in the book, and there is a good reason why I am mentioning it here again in the dinner section. Skipping your evening meal as part of an intermittent fasting routine can do wonders for your body.

In a world where our bodies are so overloaded by grains, chemicals, and environmental disturbances, there are far-reaching benefits to giving your digestive system a break from the havoc. It is a secret than many religions and spiritual leaders hold dear to their hearts.

Intermittent fasting used with coffee is a powerful method of burning fat. When your body fasts, it switches from sugar metabolism to fat metabolism, and when you add low dose caffeine to that mix, your metabolism takes it up a notch.

Now, intermittent fasting is not binge eating and then starving yourself. It is a way of timing meals for adequate fat burning. Many studies[34] have been conducted on intermittent fasting, and this "undernutrition without malnutrition" method has consistently

---

34   What The Science Says About Intermittent Fasting, http://fitness.mercola.com/sites/fitness/archive/2013/06/28/intermittent-fasting-health-benefits.aspx

improved the survival of animals with cancer. It extends their lifespan by about 30%.

- Intermittent fasting has also been found to improve the rate at which you produce human growth hormone, which is your body's "fitness" hormone.

You always have two choices: eat breakfast and lunch, and skip dinner, or eat breakfast and dinner and skip lunch.

- When you shift from eating loads of carbs to eating healthy fats like avos, eggs, coconut oil, and olive oil, your body will snap into fat burning mode. Most of your food cravings should disappear to the point where fasting takes no effort at all. In fact, fasting, for me, is just another way of saying "doing nothing."

As long as you are getting in the right calorie amount and nutrition, fasting can be a hugely beneficial method of losing fat. It suits the busy modern lifestyle by focusing on a particular window that you have to enjoy food in and then waiting for that window to come around again the next day.

- Duke University Medical Center's Dr. Stephen Freedland[35] says that intermittent fasting is as good or better than continuous calorie restriction for the human body. It improves biomarkers of disease, reduces inflammation, and curbs free radical damage. Plus, it fixes your broken hunger hormone triggers.

For me, intermittent fasting was a quick and powerful solution to my busy schedule and ever-pressing weight concerns. By the second month, I had forgotten what hunger pain even felt like unless I was particularly energetic at work that day.

---

35 Carly Harrill, What Is Intermittent Fasting (And Is It Safe?), http://naturallysavvy.com/eat/what-is-intermittent-fasting-and-is-it-safe

Sweet, Savory, and Light Dinner Pairings

Pairing specialty coffee with your dinner is an awesome way to maintain your diet while being able to eat out at a restaurant or enjoy dinner at a friend's house. You know the basic types of coffee that are involved with different food flavors, but now you need a clear idea of the flavors of coffee so that you can begin to make your own pairing decisions.

- Coffee flavor varies by region, which means that your flavor profile will depend on where you buy your coffee and how it was made.

- The coffees from Latin America (Costa Rica, Colombia, Mexico, Panama, Guatemala, and other regions of South America) are expertly balanced and are tangier than other types of bean. These are great for sweet dishes as they have medium-high acidity and have a light-medium body.

- Indonesian and other Asian coffees are uniquely earthy and woody, with many experts commenting on their floral notes and accents. This robust, full bodied coffee has a very low acidity level, which makes it perfect for high acidity meals, cheeses, and other savory dishes.

- The African and Arabian coffees are a lot more wine-like, with chocolate notes and many citrus flavors. These can also be spicy depending on the roast. They have a medium acidity and are often full bodied. I pair these coffees with light or savory meals, but I also find that some fruits fit in well here.

You should also segment your coffee according to its style. A dark espresso roast, for example, can be full bodied with low acidity—in which case it should be paired with chocolate or other sweet flavors.

French roasts work even better for nutty flavors, while Italian roasts can be exceptional with nutmeg and spices like cardamom.

You will need to test your own blends and specialty flavors by hosting some dinner parties with coffee pairings.

It is not only fun, but it is great to see the feedback for each type of coffee according to the opinions of your friends. Keep in mind that adding any extras like milk or cream are fine as long as they are used before the 5 p.m. mark.

If you cannot tolerate caffeine after dinner, choose decaf. Do not switch to tea (green and white teas are lower in caffeine), as there is almost as much caffeine in tea as there is in coffee. The myth that tea contains no caffeine is one that has caused many caffeine overdoses.

For sweet, savory, and light dinner pairings, I would stick to your single cup of coffee during the meal—which should be made up of good fats, protein, and vegetables. Your starch and carbohydrate content should be part of your nutrients. All other processed carbs do not belong on your plate.

Navigating Dinner Restaurant Foods: Coffee Please

Eating out at a modern restaurant is something of a nightmare for people that want to lose weight. This is because it is the sole goal of the restaurant to get you to enjoy your food, which means padding it with excessive portions, carbs, and other sugar-laden foods.

I learned pretty quickly that my restaurant habits were destroying my diet. I came up with a few methods of making sure that someone else's food did not impede my fat loss.

- Do not worry about portion sizes. You have no obligation to eat everything on your plate; in fact, you should stop eating when you feel full. That said, try to stick to the rule of 300 grams of meat and accompaniments.

- Leave off the bad stuff. If a meal that you love contains fries or bread or both, just tell the waiter you would like a substitution or would prefer to leave that off the plate. This will prevent you from eating it because it is in front of you.

- Request that your food be cooked in butter or olive oil. Try to stay away from other types of oil as they are very bad for your body. Never include things like sauces and dressing, as they contain a lot of sugar.

- With the demand for healthier restaurants, you can cut out a lot of risk by choosing one that serves healthy food. A recent study[36] found that working-age adults are consuming 118 fewer calories a day, than in previous years. Because of this, you can find organic, healthy restaurants with quality food in your area.

- When you select coffee off the menu at a restaurant at dinnertime, do not forget to order it black. If you cannot stomach black coffee or it is too late for you to drink regular coffee, get decaf with a dash of milk. You will still gain benefits from the existing caffeine and other supportive ingredients like disease-fighting antioxidants.

Depending on how you want to structure your Café Diet plan, you will never need to limit your eating out experiences—because the healthy lifestyle will follow you to the restaurant. If you know that your family eats out twice a week, great! Do not fast on those days, but integrate your fasting into the remainder of your week to optimize your fat loss potential.

Navigating dinner restaurant foods can be a tough one, but as long as you are vigilant and you do not overeat carbohydrates (you can eat your fill of most vegetables), you will continue to lose fat.

---

36   Melinda, Beck. Amy, Schatz, American's Eating Habits Take a Healthier Turn, Study Finds, http://online.wsj.com/news/articles/SB10001424052702304149404579323092 916490748

More than this, the following morning when you skip breakfast, the coffee will still be there preventing your hunger cravings from getting out of control.

CHAPTER 9

The Skinny on Healthy Food Choices: Snacks

"The doctor of the future will give no medication, but will interest his patients in the care of the human frame, diet and in the cause and prevention of disease."

THOMAS A EDISON

Snacks, for me, were one of the biggest habits that I had to break going into these new Café Diet cycles. For a long time, coffee and snacks were my staple, something you might identify with if eating large lunches was never really your thing.

In this chapter, I am going to take you through some important information about snacking and pairing coffee with good, healthy snacks. Then I will share a little about calorie restriction with you to simplify your diet plan.

Your Snack Food Pairing Chart

Snack foods are food items that do not need to be part of a whole meal to be delicious. At least that is how I have always defined them. You may see snack foods as a way to abate hunger or as a necessary break during your busy day.

Luckily, the most delicious snack food of all time—at least for me—is actually very good for you, and experts all over the world agree that nothing tastes better with coffee. I am talking about dark chocolate! It tops the list, which is why you can have some every week.

It feeds that "treat" center in your brain and gives you a much needed flood of dopamine because of the caffeine, light sugar, and cocoa effect. The flip side of this is that nearly every other snack food people consider delicious is baked and full of sugar.

Everything from pumpkin pie, cookies, cheesecake, and muffins has been on that snack list. These are foods that you cannot eat if you want to lose fat. Period. However, there are many other types of healthy snack foods that go well with coffee.

- When you feel like snacking on something during an off day, or breakfast was not quite enough and you need more fuel, you need to decide *how* you feel first. Do you want something sweet or something savory?
- All snacks are light, so your choices for coffee pairing involve the full spectrum. To determine which type of coffee to pair with your snack, you have to lean one way or the other first. Then, based on my previous sweet, light, and savory recommendations you, should find a good number of tasty combos.

Decide whether you want contrasting flavors or comparative flavors—and if you may want to dip your selected item. Coffee works exceptionally well with dried meat, nuts, cheeses, and sticks of raw vegetables like carrots, cucumbers, peppers, and tomatoes.

If you want to convert your daily fruit intake into a snack session, you can. Making dark chocolate dipped strawberries is an incredibly low sugar, tasty snack with coffee. Eating six or so of these will keep you going to your next meal.

Dunking and Dressing: Coffee on the Go

"Snack coffees," as I like to call them, are those restaurant or fast food coffee orders that come heavily laden with calories and frills. They are so high in sugar and extras most of the time that they can be considered snack foods.

When you are out and you want to grab a coffee, keep it simple. Go for the classic coffee recipes that I have shared with you in this book. Avoid snack coffees that have been turned into dessert drinks, iced or otherwise. They are dressed to look like a caffeine treat, but they are actually an extremely bad sugar rush.

Do not buy into the "coffee and a muffin" snack culture. Those loaded coffees are bad enough, but when you add the sugar from the muffin, it often comes to more calories than a large healthy meal would contain. And this is what we in America consider normal!

- The coffee dunking culture would have you dipping doughnuts, muffins, cookies, and other sweet treats into your coffee. This is not healthy behavior, especially if you have grabbed that coffee and snack on the go.

- When you are at a restaurant or food store, check to see if they add cream, sugar, and other chocolate-based ingredients to their coffee. The good news is that when you quit sugar, you can taste it in everything; you will know if they have added something sweet to the mix.

If you love dunking and dressing your coffee, there are ways you can still enjoy the experience without having to resort to carb-laden foods. First of all, preparation is key. You need to keep a fresh stock of food that you can eat at home or in your work fridge.

- Invest in a good coffee machine for work so that you feel like you always have access to "decadent" coffee treats without any of the unhealthy frills.

- Next to your coffee machine, there should always be some healthy dunkers and various fruit and vegetable snack items in the fridge.

The Western diet has made complex food seem simple and simple food seem complex. A muffin may be quick and easy to buy, but it is so bad for your fat problem. A tomato, on the other hand, sprinkled with some feta is a great snack, and paired with black coffee, it will zap those hunger pains away instantly—while being good for you at the same time.

I would also encourage you to explore health food stores in your area. There are lots of excellent dark chocolate-based cookies that are made without sugar and are very low calorie. If you are a natural dunker and you love to snack, make a point of preparing for it so that you can stick to your diet.

Calorie Restrictions: Knowing What to Grab

Calorie restrictions are a staple in any fat loss diet. The funny thing is that when you are aware of how many calories that you consume, it becomes part of your healthy lifestyle. When something is part of your lifestyle, it becomes a habit.

Defined, calorie restriction[37] is the dramatic reduction of calorie intake to levels that may be significantly below that for maximum growth and fertility but nutritionally sufficient for maintaining overall health.

By restricting your calories during your Café Diet cycles and then simply being aware of your calories during your off weeks, you do not have to obsess for the rest of your life about calories. The health benefits are clear—calorie restriction increases the human lifespan and mitigates disease risk.

---

37 Calorie Restriction, http://www.lef.org/protocols/lifestyle_longevity/caloric_restriction_01.htm

Instead of eating these damaging snacks when you are out, create your own versions that are healthy and fun to consume with coffee during the day. That way you can grab and eat as you like—but you will be grabbing the right food.

- Get a hold of some fresh almond flour or wheat-free, gluten-free, sugar-free flour. Bake some delicious low calorie biscotti or rusks. Eating one of these when you are hungry is a great way to boost your metabolism and avoid hunger.
- Bananas are high calorie foods, but if you love them, they make exceptional snacks. They are also full of nutrients, so you will stay fuller for longer.
- Readily available sources of protein also make for excellent coffee snacks. Think about chilled shrimp, dried meats, meatballs, and slices of cold meat that you can wrap around cheese or other veggies.
- Focus on eating raw vegetables like carrot sticks, cucumbers, and rosa tomatoes. Add some delicious nuts to the mix to liven it up.

These alternative snack food choices may not seem to go with coffee at first, but once you get rid of that sugar addiction, you will see how much better each of these items tastes. Restricting your calories is about knowing which foods are good for you and which foods hide hidden dangers for your body.

Remember, the Café Diet is only as good as your off days. If you diet for six days, lose a pound, then eat junk food for another six days, expect to gain two back. This is about reconditioning your body for improved health, not crash dieting.

Baker's Dozen: 12 Banned Foods for Your List

Which kinds of coffee compatible foods need to be struck off your snack food list? Here are the ones that you absolutely should not stomach if you want to lose fat.

- **Yogurt!** People do not realize how much sugar is added to "low-fat" yogurt. The fat content does not matter; it is the sugar that makes you gain fat. The only yogurt worth eating is Greek yogurt.

- **Trail mix.** Trail mix contains sweetened dried fruit and is laden with salt. Two small handfuls can add up to as many as 350 calories. Only eat unsalted nuts.

- **Banana chips.** They are made from banana, but they are fried in vegetable oil, so a small handful can be as much as 140 calories. The saturated fat content is also extremely bad for you.

- **Canned anything.** If it comes in a can, throw it away. There are harmful chemicals and preservatives in there that will mess with your metabolism.

- **Bagels.** One of the worst glycemic indexes around, bagels are a junk food source of instant sugar. Avoid them.

- **Doughnuts.** Known as the worst kind of food ever created, this processed, sugar-stuffed snack is a huge no-no for anyone with fat issues.

- **Margarine.** Switch to butter from today on because margarine is devastating for your body. Originally used as a method of fattening up turkeys, margarine is known as one of the worst man-made foods ever created.

- **Potato chips**. Junk food has a king, and that king is the diced, fried, and packaged potato. Trans fats will strip your body of the ability to lose fat.

- **Low calorie rice cakes**. Often a "diet" food choice, processed white rice cakes contain loads of sugar and salt even though they are low in calories.

- **Microwave popcorn.** This processed carb bomb masquerades as a healthy snack, when in fact it is loaded with trans fats and many bags are coated with chemicals to keep the popcorn from sticking to the bag. You end up eating the chemicals as well as the popcorn!

- **Baked sugar**. I call anything that has been baked and made from processed white flour, wheat, gluten, and sugar "baked sugar" because that is usually all the nutrition that you get from it.
- **Sugar and fat combos** like pizza and other baked goods with cheese or natural fat on it. Switch instead to wheat-free, gluten-free pizza bases, and watch your portions.

You may end up eating these again in your life, sure. They are around and in your face *all* the time. The problem comes in when you eat them all the time. And the modern diet forces you to pick these foods at least once or twice a day.

Shy away from these diet killers, and you will begin to condition your body for accelerated fat loss. It is tough to stick to a plan, but when it is only six days at a time, it becomes easier.

Snacking on Vitamins: Healthy Caffeine Pairing

So what sort of snacks should you be aiming for in general? The word snack is supposed to indicate a food source that gives your body nutrients that it needs because you are low on fuel. The word itself indicates that snacking in any negative form should be eliminated.

This is because modern snacking is convenient, it feeds addiction, and it is mainly for emotional comfort and wellness. The irony is that eventually these unhealthy snack foods cause depression because they mess with your body so badly.

- Smart snacking always involves some coffee. This is because you need the caffeine to reduce your hunger, and you need the healthy snack to take care of the need for more vitamins in your body.

- By keeping your calories low and your vitamin and nutrient content high, every time you snack during the Café Diet, you gain health and obliterate hunger—all while losing fat consistently.

- Snacks become more fun when they are prepared with coffee. I absolutely love strawberries dipped in dark chocolate with coffee. It is a treat, and it can be dunked and enjoyed at any time of the day.

- If you are consuming a healthy snack that contains caffeine, remember to adjust your coffee levels. It may be a good idea to switch to decaf for those snacks so that your caffeine levels do not get out of control and slow your progress.

I strongly urge you to reignite your passion for food. We all have it inside ourselves, but our busy lifestyles have buried it deep down. You know what tastes good; you just need to understand what can be done with healthier food choices.

There are many ways to overcome your sugar cravings if you plan to have them early on. Baking apples with cinnamon in the oven with a dollop of Greek yogurt can feel like a dessert. If you miss fries, experiment with butternut and zucchini chips; you can also fry kale and other veggies in olive oil for a satisfying crunch.

The goal of healthy snacking is to get in as many vitamins as you can while maintaining that low calorie threshold. You would be surprised how many excellent recipes exist for them—I certainly had no idea until I did the research.

- Test out different snacks during your various Café Diet cycles. See which ones fill you up, and detail it all in your food journal. Keeping track is a nice way of testing which foods work for you and which do not.

The hardest thing for you will be breaking your junk food habit. But you have to do that because no fat loss will happen if you do not. It confuses your hormones and really does not do anything good for your body. Keep that in mind the next time you are sitting at a drive through and have the option to order something healthy.

Navigating Café Foods: Coffee Please

One of the biggest traps for me as a roast master was coming to terms with the type of food that America sells with their coffee. Even if the coffee is incredible, the food items that surround it are not. These "cafés" have no place in the Café Diet.

- The good news is that many café's and bistros serve great egg-based breakfasts, so if you are combining breakfast and lunch, you will always find food to eat there. Ordering egg instead of wheat was the first challenge I had to face.

- The average plate of food at a café consists of a carbohydrate filled with meat, more carbohydrates on the side, and a microscopic salad. You need to shift this ideal around to become something different. The star on your plate must be the protein and the salad or vegetables, not the carb content.

- French café food like croissants, bagels, muffins, and other specialty breads must be ignored. If you are desperate for bread, get the kind made without wheat or sugar. Otherwise, it can be a learning experience to bake your own.

- Turning to exciting quiches and salads is part of traditional French café cuisine. In America, baked goods have taken over, but the skinny French still love to eat interesting salads that are brimming with nutrition. You should follow suit.

- If you walk into a café and their coffee does not seem to be simple, it is up to you to order simply. A normal cup of coffee or a cappuccino is hard to spoil. But this does not mean some places will not try—always check what goes into coffee blends.

In a perfect world, the Café Diet would strike all of the bad café foods from your diet and add nutrition and real coffee instead. It is a swap that has saved me from diabetes along with many other potential issues from my body being overweight.

Coffee started out as a healthy element in the human diet. It has become a reason to eat poorly, stay awake longer, and damage your health. If you love coffee like me, then I strongly urge you to stick to the snacks I have outlined in this chapter and remove all of those "little" devastating snacks from your life.

The truth is that I missed my junk food for the first two months. By month three, I was only snacking on healthy food. By month four, I did not even have to snack at all. It is really quite something to watch your body reshape itself. I believe everyone can do it if they are fully aware of the benefits of coffee and healthy eating.

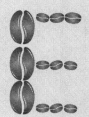

Is for Exercise: Being Full of Beans

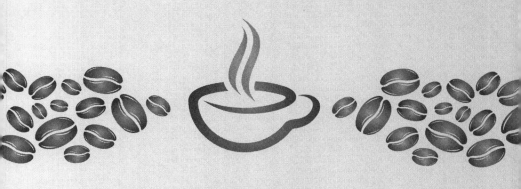

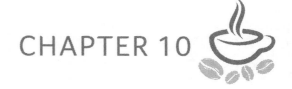

CHAPTER 10

The Mental Benefits of Coffee

"If we could give every individual the right amount of nourishment and exercise, not too little and not too much, we would have found the safest way to health."

HIPPOCRATES

In this final section of the Café Diet, I want to help you figure out where you can add more exercise to your daily life in ways that count. Coffee can be a terrific supportive tool for sourcing energy when you need it, and it has many surprising benefits too.

Even though the Café Diet was designed to work without exercise, I want to give you the opportunity to enhance your fat loss goals with some key practices. Being full of beans is about having more dynamic energy, and I can help you with that.

Physical Energy and Mental Focus

One of the largest issues with any modern diet is that it always comes with a set of stringent, close-to-impossible mental and physical barriers that you have to overcome in order for your health to improve and your fat to drop off.

Even if you can stick to a diet for a while, eventually, it has to end. I firmly believed that if I could develop a diet that ended naturally, encouraged healthy eating, and improved mental and physical energy, I could lose the excess fat that I had on my body.

The first barrier, however, was mental focus. I got stuck into the research about caffeine and mental alertness and realized that the right dose of caffeine gave me enough focus to be motivated nearly all the time.

There have been dozens of studies[38] on this, and they have found that caffeine increases selective attention and sustained attention. Selection attention is when you have to focus on a relevant stimulus. Sustained attention is when you can maintain that focus over time. With both improved after 75 mg of caffeine, this is the result.

I used the boost to focus on my eating and coffee habits, and it lasted for an optimal time of six days before I felt like I needed a break. This is why the Café Diet works in six-day cycles, because it allows for appropriate mental performance during your diet.

The physical energy that you get from coffee easily translates into mental energy when you use it to keep yourself focused on dieting. I always used to have a problem with cheating and not sticking to the diet I was on.

With the Café Diet, the cycles are so short and it is so easy to implement at any time during my normal month that it became impossible to fail. I went from being an undisciplined dieter to a master of losing fat thanks to coffee.

The Science of Motivation and Stimulation

The bottom line is that coffee contains that ever present stimulant caffeine, and that needs to be treated like a drug or a medication. Caffeine has the amazing ability to make you a lot more productive,

---

38   Mental Performance, http://www.coffeeandhealth.org/research-centre/overview/caffeine-and-mental-alertness/

engaged, and stimulated—which is perfect for those lethargic days when you are dieting and trying to lose fat.

The source of motivation[39] has long been debated, but science has helped us shed some light on it. In your brain, there are neurotransmitters that cause chemical messages to keep you alert and focused on the task you are performing. One of the main neurotransmitters is dopamine—and it plays a huge role in motivation.

Dopamine pops from one neuron to the next, interacting with your receptors inside the synapses between your neurons. There are different pathways that your neurotransmitters can take—in this instance, dopamine. It travels through the mesolimbic pathway to different places in your brain.

The main destination is the cerebral cortex, where your reward centers are. When dopamine levels increase in a certain part of your cortex, they trigger reward prediction. Your brain then actively becomes more focused and motivated because it realizes that something important is going to happen.

Dopamine is not only for pleasure; it impacts your memory, behavior, attention, and cognition as well. When you introduce a dopamine booster like caffeine into your daily diet routine, you help your brain trigger that reward center, and you instantly become more focused on the task at hand—dieting. There is real science here; I love it!

So in order to maintain your motivation for a diet, you only need two things in my opinion. First you need a diet that does not continue forever so that you can accurately have goals to work towards if your motivation and stimulation centers tend to wane as mine do.

Second you need to enhance the parts of your brain that cause motivation by stimulating them with a scientifically correct dose

39   Kevin, Lee, The Science of Motivation: Your Brain on Dopamine, http://blog.idonethis.com/post/70179626669/the-science-of-motivation-your-brain-on-dopamine

of caffeine in your morning coffee. The whole world already does this, but because of overuse, underuse, or abuse with sugar rush and sugar drop, people have forgotten that coffee can be an incredible motivator.

Motivation can be defined as the reasons that you act or behave in a specific way. For me, just the act of drinking coffee for the Café Diet prepared me physically and mentally for the day's challenges. I knew that coffee would supply the energy and focus; I just needed to do my best to keep going.

Interestingly, after the third or fourth time, I barely even noticed I was dieting. It became so natural to me that week after week I would lose fat without any effort at all. And that is why this diet needs to get out there—for unmotivated chaps like me!

The Early Morning Caffeine Curve

Let's face it; being alive in the world today is difficult. People barely get a moment's peace anymore with technology connecting everyone and making it impossible to retreat into a quiet place. The best you can hope for is an alarm sound that does not make you want to begin your day in a rampaging bad mood.

There is something called the caffeine curve that can help you clear out the cobwebs and rid yourself of the early morning grumps—and it is focused on improving your mood. Everyone wakes up tired, moody, or irritable, and depending on your food and coffee habits, this can be exacerbated at any time, for any reason.

Dieting and being in a bad mood do not go well together. Ask any man or woman that wants to shed a few pounds; it is mortally impossible when you are feeling low. Now, the caffeine curve involves knowing how much caffeine can lift your mood[40] and how much can send you careering into a fit of anxiety or agitation.

---

40   Dr Gary, Wenk, Why Does Coffee Make Us Feel So Good?, http://www. psychologytoday.com/blog/your-brain-food/201110/why-does-coffee-make-us-feel-so-good

Too much caffeine and your day will start off terribly—irritability, anger, anxiety, and headaches are just some side effects of feeling so terrible that you overuse your morning coffee fix. Too little caffeine and you may slip into withdrawal or feel foggy headed for the rest of the day. Both conditions are just not conducive to losing fat.

When you are happy and in a good mood, sticking to your diet becomes easier. The good news is that you can control the curve by getting your caffeine doses right. Here is a basic guideline to get you started.

- Have your first cup of 80 mg caffeine coffee at 7:00 a.m.
- Wait until 10:30 to have your second cup.

This is an ideal structure because it allows your brain to play with the caffeine in your system without grossly overloading it. When you consume your first cup, the caffeine will trigger a dopamine release, which contributes to feelings of wellness and euphoria.

Just when your levels start to dip, that second burst of caffeine kicks in, and you benefit from it for the next four hours at least. This takes care of your entire morning, cures those "I hate dieting" feelings that arise when you are tired and moody before work, and refocuses your mind on your goals.

Whatever you do, do not have four cups of coffee in quick succession at 7 a.m. Loads of people do this, and by 11 a.m. they are feeling three times as moody because of the crash that comes from caffeine overload. If you want to wake up and benefit from coffee like they used to do back in the old days, you need to consider its effect on your moods.

No one can be expected to fast when they are in a state of emotional distress or anxiety. From years of training, you will instantly want to reach for the first carb-rich muffin or sugar-laden treat to get that dopamine working. Pay attention to the early morning curve!

Throwing Out the Calendar: How Coffee Helps

As I mentioned before, time is always a problem for dieters. Either you have too much time, get bored, and return to your old eating habits or you have no time, get frustrated, and end up in a cycle of cheat-eating that destroys your self-esteem.

I have had to live through those horrible diets time after time, and they never did me any real good. So when I started the Café Diet, I knew that I would have to throw out the calendar and start again. Too many diet programs insist that they are "lifestyle" adjustments, and they expect you to weigh your food, count your calories, and measure your carrot sticks.

Then there are the diets that seem easy, but the food is so hard to find you have to drive across town to get those Western Himalayan yams that contain an enzyme that helps you burn fat. Again, ridiculous. There was no way that I could ever invest that much time and effort into a diet. I worked all the time, as I know you probably do too.

So I threw out the calendar and started over. Instead of building a diet around days, weeks, and months, I built the Café Diet around human rhythms and habits. *Then* I put it on a timeline. As the guinea pig, I tested different times to drink coffee, different doses, and, of course, how long I could comfortably maintain a diet plan until I wanted to give up.

The six-day, one-pound cycle was particularly effective. Instead of wishing that I would lose fat, I actively set a fat loss goal; used caffeine, techniques, and the diet to keep me on track until those six days were over; and miraculously, I would lose a pound each time. I am not talking about water weight here; I am talking about a solid pound of fat.

Coffee helps you throw out the calendar and focus on what is important—your body. It has needs, and you need to pay attention to what those needs are. That is why I want to encourage you to test your own coffee diet thresholds. You can use my testing process as a guideline, but if you are fine for eight days or 12, perhaps that is where your cycle should end.

- Notice how your body feels when you are using coffee during this fat loss process. Adjust your levels to see if it has any effect on your mood, motivation, and energy.
- Do not focus on calendar days but rather on how you feel. Record your mood in your food journal, and see if you can control it with coffee.

Coffee—when used as a medication or herb—is an exceptional way to get to know your own body. During a fat loss process like this, it is even more rewarding as you can see the rewards shortly after you have dropped the fat.

Tip! Keep a food, mood, and caffeine journal, and record your drinking times, feelings, and observations during these testing phases. Not all diets have to be so formulaic!

Curing Sleep Disorders With Coffee?

The very last thing anyone ever expects is that coffee can *help* you sleep at night. Yet new research is being conducted into this very thing. You can actually solve your sleep disorders if you know how to use coffee wisely.

In the 1980s, after years of scientists studying caffeine,[41] a breakthrough was discovered. Pharmacologists that worked with rats and mice finally proved that caffeine linked up with brain cell receptors that were sensitive to the adenosine compound—blocking their normal functioning.

---

41   Roger Downey, Health: Does Coffee Make You Sleepy?, http://www.chicagoreader.com/chicago/how-does-caffeine-affect-nervous-system-health-research/Content?oid=875717

In the right dose, adenosine reduction affects pain responses, slows reaction times, lowers attention span, and reduces appetite. The nervous system is therefore turned down instead of up. Depending on where adenosine goes, the effect can cause a surge in other neurotransmitters (dopamine for example) or a sedative effect.

These biochemists figured out that when caffeine was ingested, adenosine production stopped. But shortly after the caffeine was cleared away, adenosine production would kick back in again, causing a reaction in the body.

This is the "crash" that many people experience when they ingest low doses of caffeine. Theoretically, if you restrict your coffee consumption to mornings and the afternoon, by the time that the evening comes, your caffeine levels will wane, causing adenosine levels to rise—which will make your body naturally sleepy for the evening.

Interestingly, Narsuko Kasai, an author and nutritionist, conducted research[42] into people using caffeine for all-nighters. His theory was that drinking too many cups of coffee eventually caused drowsiness because caffeine induces trips to the bathroom. When this happens, you become more and more dehydrated and your blood moves slower in your body.

When your blood is moving slowly, it makes you tired. That is why there always comes a time during an all-nighter when you feel like passing out. The coffee has actually made you extremely tired! So drinking the right level of coffee and drinking way too much coffee can eventually exhaust you and facilitate sleep.

Beyond that, many sleep disorders can be traced back to caffeine abuse anyway. People that overuse coffee can have a cup right

---

42   Rachel Tackett, Coffee Makes You Sleepy! Nutritionist Explains The Surprising Truth About Caffeine, http://en.rocketnews24.com/2013/06/11/coffee-makes-you-sleepy-nutritionist-explains-the-surprising-truth-about-caffeine/

before they go to bed and sleep well—but it is hell getting up in the morning for them. This, once again, is a caffeine regulation issue.

If you have trouble sleeping, it might pay off to experiment with your caffeine levels and see if you can facilitate better quality sleep by limiting your intake to certain times of the day. Since I began doing it, I am convinced that the quality of my sleep is a lot better. No more waking up for no reason during the night.

Movement and Human Fat Loss Momentum

There are few things as healthy for you as a regular colon. Lucky for us, coffee has been found to stimulate colon movement, which results in evacuation of your bowels on a regular basis. Everyone is different when it comes to metabolism and bowel movements.

But when caffeine enters your system, it gets your colonic and intestinal muscles moving. This causes a process called peristalsis,[43] which is when the contents of your intestines move toward you colon.

When food moves through your colon quicker, it facilitates health and wellness—not to mention it helps boost your metabolism. This has many fat loss benefits, and it is the reason why so many people find that they need to use the facilities after their morning cuppa.

Why did you need to know this? Because fat loss is about more than losing the odd pound here and there. Even though the Café Diet attempts to give you the flexibility that you need, you should consider using it on a regular basis to gain momentum.

When I started using the Café Diet more often, my fat loss results were better than I ever could have imagined. This is because your body slips into fat burning mode, and if you can keep it there and stay motivated, you will lose more fat over time.

---

43   William McCoy, The Effects of Caffeine on Bowel Movements, http://www.livestrong.com/article/414580-the-effects-of-caffeine-on-bowel-movements/

Caffeine by its very nature causes increased human movement. It gives you all the energy you need for sharp mental focus and improved physical responses. But there are things happening beneath the surface that are beneficial as well—like your regular bowel movements. It all contributes to the marvel that is using caffeine for health.

Momentum is one of the hardest things to get right in any diet, but the bottom line is that fat loss is not a condition—it is a lifestyle choice. There are three types of people in this world. For the majority of people, they gain fat every year because of stress, age, and bad food choices.

Then there are those that lose weight all the time because they yo-yo diet. Gaining and losing, gaining and losing—it is a horrible way to live. Finally, the third kind of person loses all of their weight and then maintains that fat loss with a healthy diet.

I fit into that third category, and I want you to fit into it too. That is why I hope you use the Café Diet methods to restructure your eating patterns and your coffee habits for long-term benefits. The short-term rewards are great, but the long-term ones are better.

Use caffeine to enhance your mental and physical state and to control your moods. Striking the right balance means that you will have finally harnessed the power of one of the healthiest stimulants in the world. The benefits will blow your mind.

CHAPTER 11

Coffee Fueled Exercise for Life

"If you always put limits on everything you do, physical or anything else, it will spread into your work and into your life. There are no limits. There are only plateaus; and you must not stay there, you must go beyond them."

BRUCE LEE

As I mentioned at the beginning of this final section, coffee has some pretty incredible benefits if you learn how to use it in conjunction with exercise. There are many "lazy" ways to take advantage of this that I will share with you here.

Tweaking your performance is all about timing, doses, and stress release. Hopefully, the exercise that you choose will give you all the benefits that my Aikido training gave me. It is the step up that you need when your diet has been sorted out.

The Benefits of Pre-Workout Coffee

When I was deep into my Café Diet cycles, I realized that I had enough energy to expend on some kind of physical activity outside of work. I wanted to enhance my mental, emotional, and physical aspects, so I looked for a sport that would concentrate on these things.

I found Aikido, and it instantly sparked my interest. I was never a big fan of punching and kicking, so I wanted something different. Aikido was a great, non-violent martial art that appealed to me. Later, when I went through the previous months in my mind, I realized that it added a third dimension to my weight loss goals.

It was something new and enjoyable in my life, and I think people vastly underestimate the value that this has. It helped distract me from hunger and gave me something to look forward to that was completely outside of my comfort zone.

Best of all, it allowed me to expend all of that energy I was getting from caffeine in a way that facilitated even more fat loss. The movement was great, and I learned a valuable lesson. While lots of diet plans tell you to lose fat and be happy, I came to realize that you have to be happy to lose fat. They have it back to front!

There are so many benefits to using coffee before you work out or exercise. More than two-thirds of about 20,680 Olympic athletes[44] were found to have caffeine in their urine—with the highest amounts being for triathletes, cyclists, and rowers. Clearly, the energy and endurance benefits of caffeine have serious value.

- Caffeine makes you feel like you have more energy.
- Caffeine helps you endure physical exercise.
- Caffeine assists in muscle growth and overall wellness.
- Caffeine reduces muscle pain from exercise.
- Caffeine improves precision and accuracy in sport.
- Caffeine helps your body burn more fat.

How Long Does a Coffee High Last?

A good caffeine high or "buzz" depends on the type of coffee that

---

44 Gretchen, Reynolds, How Coffee Can Galvanize Your Workout, http://well.blogs.nytimes.com/2011/12/14/how-coffee-can-galvanize-your-workout/?_php=true&_type=blogs&_r=0

you are drinking and the rate at which you have consumed it. Assuming that you regulate your caffeine levels, drinking a normal cup of coffee will have this effect.

- The more caffeine that you consume, the more the stimulant effect will be exacerbated. Keep this in mind when measuring your pre-workout dose.

- You will begin to feel the effects of coffee within 15 minutes.[45] It takes about 45 minutes for those effects to be full blown in your system.

- Caffeine has a half-life of about four to six hours. This means that you will be buzzing for at least two hours, and it takes four to six hours for that effect to reduce by half. This gives you plenty of time to enjoy your morning workout.

- If you dose yourself with 300 mg of caffeine for a power boost at 6 a.m., by 12 a.m. you will still have 150 mg of caffeine in your bloodstream.

- If you smoke, the half-life of caffeine is only three hours—which is why so many chain smokers are also very heavy coffee drinkers.

For maximum physical benefits, you will need to drink your cup of coffee an hour before your workout or your exercise routine. The "high" from coffee may work out of your system faster depending on the intensity of your exercise.

Coffee highs are great workout tools because they quickly and safely improve your energy levels, your endurance, and your ability to push yourself hard when it counts. I only really began to appreciate the power of caffeine when I did Aikido.

After the first month, I had so much energy I was ready for every single day. The coffee helped me get through that transition

---

45   Gina, Reggio, How Long Does Coffee Stay in Your System, http://www.livestrong.com/article/272782-how-long-does-coffee-caffeine-stay-in-your-system/

period when you are unfit, tired, moody, and have no motivation to exercise at all.

- The mental effects of caffeine are lasting. This is because they transform into the mental benefits of exercise once you get through those first few grueling classes.
- The physical effects of caffeine are also lasting. This is because you gain muscle and reshape really quickly when you are using caffeine to reshape and exercise. I was surprised by how quickly I managed to grow muscle.

Putting Together Your Exercise Schedule

When I chose Aikido, I did so because I wanted to learn something new and fun, and I was not interested in anything too complex, expensive, or team-based. Like me, you will need to decide where your interests lie and which exercises could catapult you ahead of your own fat loss goals.

The real power of caffeine kicks in when you exercise on it. I recommend that you do at least one type of exercise or activity along with your diet plan. This can be something that you can do at home, or it can be a class.

The most important thing is that you find something you enjoy. There is no point doing any kind of exercise that you hate doing, because you will not do it for long. If you have old exercise equipment at home, think of new ways to make your routine fun.

- If rowing or running on a treadmill is too boring for you, use technology to spice it up. There are trail runs that you can watch on YouTube, audio books you can listen to for self-development, or comedy shows that will lighten your day.
- If you have a cycle or elliptical trainer at home, jump on with some energetic music. You can go to dozens of different sites

online for music that has been specially made for gym spin classes, but you can do at home.

- If you love the outdoors but are not a huge fan of running, get your friends together and go on hikes. This will improve your fitness levels, get in some social time, and give you the opportunity to reconnect with nature.

- Make your exercise time an opportunity to track your fat loss and figure out new ways to improve your performance. Get a wearable device that tracks your vitals, steps, and fitness level, and turn exercising into a game.

The sad reality is that most people that need to lose weight have a two-headed problem. They are eating badly, and they are not exercising enough. This is mainly due to demanding work hours, busy family lives, and almost no time for anything else.

The good news is that when you start to use caffeine in your exercise routines, you will quickly recover from that perpetual exhaustion that you feel—I did! Once you get your blood flowing and your legs moving, the natural energy that results is heady.

Assemble a 30-minute exercise plan that kicks in at least three times a week. Anyone and everyone I have ever met can spare an hour and a half a week for personal fitness and fat loss. You will love it so much that soon it will be a daily routine.

Cardio and Coffee: What You Need to Know

If you are into the more cardio-based sports like running, swimming, cycling, and rowing, then there are some things that you will need to know about your coffee levels. Tweaking the effects of caffeine in your body is always a good idea, as everyone is different.

- Each morning when you wake up you should first have a cup of black coffee an hour before your workout.

- Work out for at least 30 minutes, but keep in mind that you can increase this to two hours if you want to later on because caffeine lasts.
- Once you are finished exercising, you should eat your large, tasty breakfast. Your body will be in a fat burning state and will quickly metabolize your breakfast, giving you a power boost for the day.
- Between 10:30 and 12:30 you should have your second cup of coffee. This will reignite your fat burning processes and raise your caffeine levels again.

There is much controversy over whether or not you should or should not drink a cup of coffee post-workout. I think that to stay safe, you should remain coffee free until the designated time—two hours after your workout.

This is to keep the caffeine levels in your body stable and not too high, as the caffeine may increase your cortisol levels and will cause visceral fat to form across your belly if you are not careful. Of course, there is no evidence that this will happen to you—especially if you work out fairly often and are following the Café Diet plan.

A recent Canadian study[46] showed the effect of caffeine on running times and levels of exhaustion. There were nine men who were involved in five trials. An hour before each run, the men took either a caffeine capsule, a placebo, regular coffee, or decaf with added caffeine.

The results showed that caffeine increased the men's performance by up to 10 times. It all depends on the dose that you take and the condition that you are in. As you become more fit, your caffeine dose will push you further and harder, resulting in more fat loss.

Coffee and caffeine have been proven to prolong endurance,

---

46   The Effects of Caffeine on Exercise Performance, https://www.weightlossresources.co.uk/exercise/workouts/caffeine-performance.htm

which is great for cardio exercises that need to either increase in intensity or duration. You can adjust yours according to your fitness level and how well your coffee works.

Weight Training and Caffeine: The Facts

Weight training is an excellent strength-based exercise that may suit your lifestyle better than general cardio does. In fact, weight training helps you build more muscle, which actually improves your fat loss potential.

The great thing is that caffeine directly affects the muscles in your body. A study by the Society for Experimental Biology[47] determined that caffeine boosts power in older muscles. Older people should actually drink coffee to improve their muscle strength! The principles are the same for younger people too.

Caffeine helps muscles produce more force, which actively leads to improved muscle growth over time. This is great because it reduces your injury potential if you are a little past the age of 45, like I am. Aging muscle needs to be strong, but it is hard getting there.

- Drinking a cup of coffee or two before you weight train will help you lift heavier weights. That means your muscles will get bigger.
- The caffeine in coffee will keep you pushing yourself harder during high intensity reps, which will also contribute to muscle growth and development.
- Because you work harder on caffeine, all of the benefits of weight training become amplified. For someone with pre-diabetes or type 2 diabetes, this means having greater surface area for your insulin receptors, which will help regulate your insulin.

---

47   Joshua Wortman, Caffeine Enhances Muscle Performance, http://breakingmuscle.com/nutrition/caffeine-enhances-muscle-performance

- According to The American Physiological Society,[48] you should work out, eat some carbohydrates, and then drink a few cups of coffee. Glycogen is needed to build muscle, and when you eat carbs and drink coffee immediately after your workout (three hours later), the caffeine will facilitate muscle growth from the carbs.

- It is a good idea to include some low carb foods inside your egg breakfast if you are going to weight train. I suggest butternut, broccoli, cauliflower, or sweet potato. The caffeine in your system will metabolize these and help your muscles grow.

A good solid weight training workout is about 25 minutes long and focuses more on the intensity of the reps than the number of reps. Start by lifting until you get muscle fatigue, then record your times. Slowly, they will improve—then rapidly!

Coffee and Sport: Cool Beans

If cardio exercise and weight training at home is not your thing, what remains is to take a class or to find a sport that you can enjoy at least twice a week. Often sport is a way of exercising with other people and having fun at the same time.

There have been some incredible studies into precision sports like soccer and how coffee reduces reaction time and improves performance. In a recent Taekwondo study,[49] the researchers found that participants in the test group had quicker reactions times than the previous round when they did not have caffeine in their bodies.

Caffeine can make you more accurate at a sport, give you greater endurance, and give you a great boost of energy when you need to

---

48 Donna Krupa, Post-Exercise Caffeine Helps Muscles Refuel, http://www.the-aps.org/mm/hp/Audiences/Public-Press/For-the-Press/releases/Archive/08/24.html
49 Victor GF Santos, Caffeine Reduces Reaction Time and Improves Performance in Simulated Content of Taekwondo, http://www.ncbi.nlm.nih.gov/pmc/articles/PMC3942723/

relieve some stress. If you are going to join a team or do a sport, I suggest the following:

- Try to find a morning sport or class like yoga that works on the muscles if you enjoy slow-paced exercise or team-based sports like soccer if you enjoy fast-paced sports with lots of people competing against each other.

- If you cannot find a morning class, an evening one is fine—but you will have to watch your caffeine levels. Drinking a cup of coffee or two before your sport is fine because the energy will be used. By the time you get home from your class, you should be relaxed and ready for a peaceful night's sleep.

- Do not get encouraged to start taking caffeine supplements for any reason, as they will throw off your fat loss goals. A dance class or regular trips to the golf course can do wonders for a body that is trying to slim down.

Coffee and sport have gone together for as long as they have been around. The trick is to enjoy what you do, or you will not continue doing it. I have met people that have hated sport their whole lives only to discover one that they love in their fifties.

There are so many in this world, so if you enjoy surfing, climbing, cricket, football, extreme Frisbee—whatever attracts you—go and check it out! There are also various levels of competency. You may want to join a team that does not compete but just has friendly games with other clubs for no-pressure fun.

CHAPTER 12

Fat Loss Maintenance With Coffee

"Nothing can stop the man with the right mental attitude from achieving his goal; nothing on earth can help the man with the wrong mental attitude."

THOMAS JEFFERSON

In this final chapter, I want to run through some important points about keeping off the fat that you lose with the Café Diet. After all, there is no reason to diet if your fat is going to continue to jump back onto your body again.

Fat loss maintenance is a critical element of the Café Diet, and it involves some lifestyle changes on your part. On the whole, the diet is easy—all it takes is choice. If you can make the right choice, then you can lose all of your fat.

Athletic Performance and the Café Diet

The American College of Sports Medicine mentioned a recent study[50] that indicates ingesting 3–9 mg of caffeine per kilogram of

---

50   Caffeine and Exercise Performance, http://www.acsm.org/docs/current-comments/caffeineandexercise.pdf

body weight one hour before you exercise does improve running and cycling performance in a lab environment.

Many athletes use caffeine when they are training to boost their performance. Whether you are a pro or not does not matter; caffeine will give you that little something extra when you need it. Once you sort out your caffeine and sugar levels, you will finally begin to feel the real effects of caffeine.

That means within an hour of drinking a fresh cup of coffee before you exercise, you will feel more energized to do it. I never understood what people were talking about until I had a handle on my levels. Seriously, there is a noticeable increase in energy when you are particular about the coffee that you drink.

For people like me who suffered from lack of motivation for most of my life, there is now some serious science behind a second option. Once you have fixed your will to exercise, all that remains is having the energy to do so.

A lot of the time people that want to get fit cannot start properly because they are so darn exhausted. Work, a new diet, and all the other responsibilities sneak in, and exercise becomes the area where the least energy is invested.

And this is a shame because the more you exercise, the more you want to exercise. It only takes that first month or two to get you into the habit and for the movement to eventually replenish your lost energy stores.

To this day if I feel too tired to exercise, I immediately go and make a cup of coffee. Within an hour I feel noticeably better, and off I go. It really does help fix that energy deficit that your average day creates. There is nothing better than that feeling you get after you have exercised once you are more fit. It turns from exhaustion into elation.

The Perfect Weight to Caffeine Ratio

There is a lot to learn about using caffeine according to your weight. The athletes in the world all use caffeine according to their total body mass. The substance itself actually makes a difference to your workout on multiple levels.

The impact is so vast that caffeine was once on the list of banned stimulants for the Olympic Games. Just eight cups of coffee is enough to provoke a ban from the Olympic committee. Even though caffeine is not banned anymore, it is still screened in tests.

What caffeine does is it improves your blood flow from the heart to the rest of your body. It smashes fatigue and increases the amount of adrenaline in your body. The right things rush to your muscles, and you are ready to go.

So how much caffeine should you drink to tap into your peak performance levels? I am going to outline that for you here.

- If you exercise in the morning, you should begin with one cup of coffee regardless of your weight to test the effects once you have your levels under control.

- A good two to three milligrams per two lbs thereafter will do the trick, or the equivalent of and a 176lb / 80 kilo individual drinking two to three cups of coffee. If you are going to consume two cups of coffee in the morning, that leaves you with only one during the day.

- You should drink the two cups an hour before you work out, as many studies have indicated. Moderate doses are the only doses that work. Do not flood your system with caffeine for any reason, or you will end up crashing hard afterwards.

- Caffeine in coffee is like any other drug—if you drink too much of it, eventually a tolerance is going to form. The last thing you want is for your tolerance to push you into the red zone (400 mg or more). Keep it low so that you can lose fat, build muscle, and exercise like a champion.

- Caffeine works on two levels: it gives you more endurance so that you can exercise for longer, and it improves performance of quick-burst exercise, giving you more power when you need it.

Here is a quick caffeine index for your weight:

330 lb /150 kilos	3 cups of coffee
264 lb /120 kilos	3 cups of coffee
198 lb / 90 kilos	2 cups of coffee
154 lb / 70 kilos	1–2 cups of coffee
110 lb / 50 kilos	1–2 cups of coffee

Tracking Fat Loss Using Natural Coffee

There is a very straightforward method that I used to discover coffee's importance to my exercise and fat loss goals. Some people say that coffee is not relevant and that making these diet changes will work just as well.

The only problem with that is that it does not. That is why it is called the Café Diet, because coffee is central to the fat loss process. I tested it on myself to see what kind of difference it made. You can do the same thing if you want to see if it works.

- Begin the Café Diet as usual, and write down all of your stats beforehand. Include what you weigh and what you want to weigh.
- You cannot run this test in the first two months, as accelerated fat loss always happens in the beginning, which could skew the results.
- When you are two months in and your caffeine levels have

been steadily helping you lose fat, record your metrics on that final week.

- Then, when the next Café Diet cycle comes along, stop drinking coffee altogether. You will not have a lot of withdrawal because your coffee levels are stable.

- For the next six-day cycle, record your metrics meticulously. Take note of how you feel, how often you exercise, when you eat, and why. Compare it to your previous cycle.

When I tracked my fat loss this way, I realized that caffeine was literally plugging those little holes that other diets overlook. Off coffee I was more tired, I was moodier, I was less dynamic at work, and I exercised less. More to the point, I lost less fat that week on a system that has been quite predictable.

Now, this is not a scientific experiment, and my physiology is different to yours anyway. But I am quite confident that if you run this little test, you will see how much difference it really makes. Get back on the caffeine for the next cycle, and record how you feel.

There is nothing like not going near a cup of coffee or any caffeine and then tasting that awesome coffee and experiencing that boost again. Coffee has been the fat loss supporter that I always needed.

It gives me energy, which helps me stay focused and motivated. It keeps my hunger at bay, which keeps me from cheating on the diet. It even helps improve my performance when I exercise so that I get fitter quicker.

And that is why I wanted to write this book so badly. Day after day I see people online who struggle with fat loss because of these *same* issues. There is no trick, no gimmick—nothing. Simply adjust your levels, correct your diet and fat will fall away.

The World's Most Important Beverage: Drink Up

There are lots of reasons to enjoy coffee every single day. It is the world's most important beverage and a sheer delight to use in low doses. It is completely safe, and it adds to the health and longevity of your life.

- Coffee makes you feel less tired and actively increases your energy levels because of caffeine, the active ingredient.
- Coffee makes you smarter by enhancing your brain function.[51] Once you drink coffee, the caffeine enters your bloodstream and, eventually, your brain. When it is in your brain, it blocks an inhibitor called adenosine. This naturally increases the production of other neurotransmitters like dopamine and norepinephrine. Your neurons fire faster, and your brain function improves!
- Coffee is a natural fat burner. Caffeine, the active ingredient, has been proven to boost your metabolic rate,[52] and under the right circumstances, you will burn more fat—as much as 10%, in fact, depending on your weight.
- Coffee lowers your risk for type 2 diabetes. There are dozens of studies[53] supporting the fact that coffee in low doses keeps diabetes at bay.
- Coffee is bursting with essential nutrients that are great for your body. Just one little cup of coffee and you will ingest riboflavin (B12), manganese, potassium, niacin, magnesium, and pantothenic acid (B5).
- Coffee loves to improve your physical performance. It can be fairly significant, but you will have to test how far it takes you.

51   AL McCall, Blood-Brain Barrier Transport of Caffeine: Dose-Related Restriction of Adenine Transport, http://www.sciencedirect.com/science/article/pii/0024320582907159
52   Kevin Acheson, Metabolic Effects of Caffeine in Humans: Lipid Oxidation or Futile Cycling?, http://ajcn.nutrition.org/content/79/1/40.full.pdf+html
53   Rob van Dam, Coffee Consumption and Risk of Type 2 Diabetes Mellitus, http://www.sciencedirect.com/science/article/pii/S014067360211436X

Aside from these amazing health benefits, studies have also been conducted to investigate how coffee protects from Alzheimer's disease and dementia, and it reduces a person's risk of getting Parkinson's disease as well. A few other pleasant side effects of enjoying coffee in the right doses include protection against liver issues and depression.

It is no wonder that coffee is the largest source of antioxidants in the Western diet today. As long as you remain below that 400 mg threshold, you are perfect. Any more than that and the benefits can swing into some pretty severe negative side effects.

Coffee is hands down the most important beverage in the world today. Scientists are still uncovering new things about the bean centuries after its discovery. I am sure that in the future, coffee will become an even more prominent beverage in society.

10 Weird Facts About Coffee

Now that we have taken a look at all of coffee's wonderful benefits, it is time to take an even closer look at coffee's eccentricities. Just when you think you know everything there is to know about coffee, more weird facts arise. I will share them with you here.

1. A single espresso does not have more caffeine in it than a normal cup of coffee. This is a common myth! Due to serving sizes, espresso usually has about a third the amount of caffeine in it.

2. Caffeine can kill you but only if you consume more than 100 cups of it, which is impossible. People have died from caffeine-related heart attacks however.

3. Coffee is a fruit. Or more accurately, it is the seed in the coffee berry that is then dried and roasted into the coffee we love today. Drinking a cup of coffee is the same as drinking a very specialist type of fruit drink!

4. Java and Mocha are both names of ports. The coffee bean had such a huge impact when it first arrived that both types of coffee were named after the ports they came from.

5. Coffee beans are a renewable source of energy. Because the beans are combustible, they may one day replace fossil fuels as our main source of energy. In 2011 a car was created that ran on nothing but coffee beans.[54]

6. People in New York love coffee so much that they drink about seven times more of it than any other city on earth. New York City is the coffee capital of the world.

7. The Turkish community loved coffee so much that once upon a time, if a husband did not provide his wife with coffee, legally she could file for divorce. The law has since changed, but it says a lot about how important coffee is in their culture.

8. Coffee is the reason why developing countries can develop! Most coffee farming happens in developing nations, which then sell it to developed nations, moving money between the two. Coffee builds economies!

9. Coffee called Kopi Luwak is the world's most expensive coffee at about $600 per pound. It is created on wild cat farms in Sumatra—the cats are fed coffee beans, and when they are excreted, the beans are turned into coffee.

10. The world record for the most cups of coffee ever consumed was by a coffee lover who drank 82 cups in seven hours. He probably did not sleep for several days.

The rich culture that has inspired such incredible stories is all part of coffee's appeal. The more you research, the deeper it goes. Coffee has touched the lives of everyone and everything. It is truly a beverage for the people.

---

54   Sebastian Anthony, British Coffee-Powered Car Breaks World Record, http://www.extremetech.com/extreme/97287-british-coffee-powered-car-breaks-world-record

Few things are as magical in life as standing in an open field, watching the sun rise with a cup of coffee in your hands. It gives you time to stop, be present, and experience the elation that comes from coffee indulgence.

When you learn to control your caffeine levels, you will become excited about coffee again. I urge you to invest in a brand or blend that is a cut above your normal grocery store stuff. Stick to carefully made blends or straight strains. Never allow your coffee to just be something that gives you a caffeine boost.

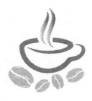

Conclusion

The Café Diet is very much like a good cup of coffee. It fits into your life and makes everything better. From losing fat to getting fitter and the changes inside, you will be much healthier. The benefits are transferred over to you when you decide to become a Café Diet advocate.

The science of fat loss has always been there, but those little problems that prevent you from losing the weight have never had any real solutions. I have walked you through my own experiences and research on coffee.

This diet proves that it is not just fat loss that matters but health. I became so much healthier after following this diet that my cholesterol and triglyceride levels normalized and my fasting blood sugar level dropped, which rapidly improved my insulin sensitivity—reversing my risk for contracting type 2 diabetes! Diabetes is a killer, and I sidestepped it.

This showed me that the Café Diet was more about gaining my life back than losing fat. It is a big plan with big benefits, and that is why I felt compelled to share it with the world.

Now you know exactly how to regulate your caffeine levels, how to assemble your plan, and how to keep the fat off forever. All it takes is a goal and an infusion of coffee to get it right! I hope the Café Diet has helped you sort out some of your issues with fat and food.

When I first started, I never believed that one day my experience would be a book. But I am so glad that I embraced it and had the courage to share this knowledge. I changed my life because of coffee, or perhaps coffee was always destined to change yours.

If you picked up this book and read it, you are now equipped with the tools you need to lose fat when you need to. It is a perfect plan for anyone that does not have time for much exercise and definitely does not have time to be tired all day from dieting and physical exertion. You will not feel either of those things once you get into this diet.

As I mentioned before, I am just a roast master with a dream. Coffee helped me lose my excess fat, and I know that it can help you lose yours too using science, discipline, and delicious coffee. Before you know it, you will feel healthier and be happier than you have been in years.

Your body will reshape itself, and fat will become a distant memory. If, like me, you have always been a little overweight, just a few cycles of the Café Diet will fix that. It all begins with a nice low caffeine cup.

Cheers!
Béla Csepregi

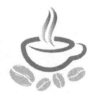

References

Chapter 1

King, Alexander, Welcome to the Quote Garden, http://www.quotegarden.com/coffee.html

Cafestol, http://en.wikipedia.org/wiki/Cafestol

Coffee, Jason, 18 Amazing Coffee Quotes, http://coffeecupnews.org/coffee-quotes/

International Coffee Organization, Frequently Asked Questions, http://www.ico.org/show_faq.asp?show=35

Coffee Drinking Statistics, http://www.statisticbrain.com/coffee-drinking-statistics/

What Is Coffee? http://www.ncausa.org/i4a/pages/index.cfm?pageID=67

Berardi, John, Coffee: Your Poison or Your Medicine?, http://www.huffingtonpost.com/john-berardi-phd/coffee-health-benefits_b_3881377.html

Coffee Farming & Processing, http://www.zecuppa.com/coffeeterms-farming-processing.htm

The Reunion Island Coffee Café, http://www.reunionislandcoffee.com/Learn-About-Coffee-Farming-s/33.htm

Kew Royal Botanic Gardens, Coffea Arabica (Arabica Coffee), http://

www.kew.org/science-conservation/plants-fungi/coffea-arabica-arabica-coffee

Bengis RO, Anderson RJ, The Chemistry of the Coffee-Bean: 1. Concerning the Unsaponifiable Matter of the Coffee-Bean Oil. Preparation And Properties of Kahweol, http://www.jbc.org/content/97/1/99.full.pdf

Urgent, Robert, Schulz, Angela GM, Effects of Cafestol And Kahweol From Coffee Grounds on Serum Lipids and Serun Liver Enzymes In Humans, http://ajcn.nutrition.org/content/61/1/149.full.pdf

Food Info, Kahweol and Cafestol, http://www.food-info.net/uk/products/coffee/kahweol.htm

Kahweol, http://en.wikipedia.org/wiki/Kahweol

Zurow, Lydia, How Coffee Influenced the Course of History, http://www.npr.org/blogs/thesalt/2013/04/24/178625554/how-coffee-influenced-the-course-of-history

International Coffee Organization, The Story of Coffee, http://www.ico.org/coffee_story.asp

National Geographic, Beyond the Buzz, http://www.nationalgeographic.com/coffee/ax/frame.html

Etymology First Uses of Coffee, http://www.thecoffeecoach.in/2011/04/etymology-first-uses-of-coffee/

List of Coffee Drinks, http://coffee.wikia.com/wiki/List_of_coffee_drinks

The Love of Coffee Throughout History, Famous Coffee Lovers, http://www.podmerchant.com/newsletter/PC044-famous-coffee-lovers-lucaffe-messico.html

Ferdman, Roberto A, Where the World's Biggest Coffee Drinkers Live, http://qz.com/166983/where-the-worlds-biggest-coffee-drinkers-live/

Bowers, Ben, I'll Take Mine…How 16 Men of Note Take Their Coffee, http://gearpatrol.com/2013/02/27/how-fifteen-men-of-note-take-their-coffee/#danlyons

Chapter 2

Lynch, David, Coffee Quotes, http://www.brainyquote.com/quotes/keywords/coffee_2.html

Boyles, Salynn, Drinking Coffee May Extend Life, http://www.webmd.com/heart/news/20080616/drinking-coffee-may-extend-life

Aborn, Shana, The Healing Power of Coffee, http://www.drozner.com/uploads/3/0/1/1/3011688/hap_-_health_radar_nov_2012.pdf

The Healing Powers of Coffee, http://www.annlouise.com/blog/2011/08/02/the-healing-powers-of-coffee/

Ferraro, Diane, Coffee and Your Health: Healing Benefits of Coffee, http://imperfectwomen.com/coffee-and-your-health-healing-benefits-of-coffee/

Sinatra, Stephen, Dr, The Health Benefits of Drinking Coffee, http://www.drsinatra.com/the-health-benefits-of-drinking-coffee

Lipschitz, David, Dr, Drinking More Coffee Can Extend Life: Who Knew? http://www.creators.com/health/david-lipschitz-lifelong-health/drinking-more-coffee-can-extend-life-who-knew.html

Barclay, Laurie, MD, The Disease-Fighting Power of Polyphenols, https://www.lef.org/magazine/mag2008/feb2008_The-Disease-Fighting-Power-Of-Polyphenols_01.htm

Scalbert, Augustin, Johnson, Ian T, Saltmarsh, Mike, Polyphenols: Antioxidants and Beyond 1'2'3, http://ajcn.nutrition.org/content/81/1/215S.full

The Healthful Benefits of Polyphenols, http://www.goodhealth.com.au/271/nutrition/the-healthful-benefits-of-polyphenols/

Sifferlin, Alexandra, The Truth About Antioxidants, http://healthland.time.com/2013/08/06/the-truth-about-antioxidants/

Antioxidants: Beyond the Hype, http://www.hsph.harvard.edu/nutritionsource/antioxidants/

Arendash, GW, Cao, C, Caffeine and Coffee as Therapeutics Against Alzheimer's Disease, http://www.ncbi.nlm.nih.gov/pubmed/20182037

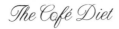

Cao, Chuanhai, PhD, Arendash, Gary, PhD, USF Study: Mystery Ingredient in Coffee Boosts Protection Against Alzheimer's Disease, http://hscweb3.hsc.usf.edu/health/now/?p=19816

Hyman, Mark, MD, Ten Reasons to Quit Your Coffee! http://drhyman.com/blog/2012/06/13/ten-reasons-to-quit-your-coffee/

Can Stress Make You Fat? http://www.fitday.com/fitness-articles/fitness/can-stress-make-you-fat.html#b

Gottfried, Sara, MD, Cortisol Switcharoo: How the Main Stress Hormone Makes You Fat And Angry, http://www.huffingtonpost.com/sara-gottfried-md/cortisol_b_1589670.html

Kosner, Anthony, Wing, Why the Best Time to Drink Coffee Is Not First Thing in the Morning, http://www.forbes.com/sites/anthonykosner/2014/01/05/why-the-best-time-to-drink-coffee-is-not-first-thing-in-the-orning/http://www.ncbi.nlm.nih.gov/pmc/articles/PMC2257922/

MacDougall, Caroline, Six Tips to Reduce the Stress Hormone, Cortisol, http://teeccino.com/building_optimal_health/148/Six-Tips-To-Reduce-The-Stress-Hormone,-Cortisol.html

Caffeine and Mental Alertness – Part 2, http://www.coffeeandhealth.org/research-centre/overview/caffeine-and-mental-alertness-part-2/

Coffee – Mental Performance and Wellness, http://www.medindia.net/patients/lifestyleandwellness/coffee-caffeine-decaf-health-mental-performance-wellness.htm

Johnson-Koslow, Marilyn, Kritz-Silverstein, Donna, Barrett-Connor, Elizabeth, Morton, Deborah, Coffee Consumption and Cognitive Function Among Older Adults, http://aje.oxfordjournals.org/content/156/9/842.full

Coffee Health Benefits: Coffee May Protect Against Disease, http://www.health.harvard.edu/press_releases/coffee_health_benefits

Hellmich, Nanci, Eating Too Much Added Sugar May Be Killing You, http://www.usatoday.com/story/news/nation/2014/02/03/added-sugars-heart-disease-death/5183799/

Appleton, Nancy, PhD, Jacobs, GN, 141 Reasons Sugar Ruins Your

Health, http://nancyappleton.com/141-reasons-sugar-ruins-your-health/

Do You Ruin Your Coffee? Don't Waste Your Coffee's Health Benefits, http://www.odacremcoffee.com/blog/keep-your-coffee-healthy/

Mercola, Dr, Mounting Evidence Suggests Coffee May Actually Have Therapeutic Health Benefits, http://articles.mercola.com/sites/articles/archive/2012/09/16/coffee-health-benefits.aspx

Moawad, Heidi, Dr, Signs and Symptoms of Caffeine Intolerance, http://www.livestrong.com/article/538019-signs-symptoms-of-caffeine-intolerance/

Borelli, Lizette, What's The Best Time to Drink Coffee? The Hour Matters Because Cortisol Cycle Influences Caffeine Effectiveness, http://www.medicaldaily.com/whats-best-time-drink-coffee-hour-matters-because-cortisol-cycle-influences-caffeine-effectiveness

Miller, Steven, PhD, The Best Time for Your Coffee, http://neurosciencedc.blogspot.com.au/2013/10/the-best-time-for-your-coffee.html

Chapter 3

Camus, Albert, Quotes About Coffee, http://www.goodreads.com/quotes/tag/coffee

Hartel, Kari, RD, LD, The Skinny on Losing Weight With Green Coffee Beans, http://www.fitday.com/fitness-articles/nutrition/the-skinny-on-losing-weight-with-green-coffee-beans.html#b

Salzberg, Steven, Dr. Oz Tries to Do Science: The Green Coffee Bean Experiment, http://www.forbes.com/sites/stevensalzberg/2013/09/09/dr-oz-tries-to-do-science/

Find a Vitamin or Supplement – Green Coffee,

http://www.webmd.com/vitamins-supplements/ingredientmono-1264-GREEN%20COFFEE.aspx?activeIngredientId=1264&activeIngredientName=GREEN%20COFFEE

Moderate Coffee Consumption Won't Cause Dehydration, Study Finds, http://www.huffingtonpost.com/2014/01/09/coffee-dehydration-moderate-consumption_n_4568059.html

O'Connor, Anahad, The Claim: Caffeine Causes Dehydration, http://www.nytimes.com/2008/03/04/health/nutrition/04real.html?_r=0

Aubrey, Allison, Coffee Myth-Busting: Cup of Joe May Help Hydration and Memory, http://www.npr.org/blogs/thesalt/2014/01/13/262175623/coffee-myth-busting-cup-of-joe-may-help-hydration-and-memory

Gunnars, Kris, Can Coffee Increase Your Metabolism and Help You Burn Fat?, http://authoritynutrition.com/coffee-increase-metabolism/

Smatresk, Neal J, How Does Caffeine Affect the Body, http://www.scientificamerican.com/article/how-does-caffeine-affect/

Miller, Steve, PhD, The Best Time to Drink Coffee According to Science, http://en.ilovecoffee.jp/posts/view/110

Kosner, Anthony, Wing, Why the Best Time to Drink Coffee Is Not First Thing in the Morning, http://www.forbes.com/sites/anthonykosner/2014/01/05/why-the-best-time-to-drink-coffee-is-not-first-thing-in-the-morning/

Are Multiple Cups of Coffee a Day Bad for Your Health? http://www.fitday.com/fitness-articles/nutrition/healthy-eating/are-multiple-cups-of-coffee-a-day-bad-for-your-health.html#b

Oatman, Maddie, 9 Things You Should Know About Your Caffeine Habit, http://www.motherjones.com/environment/2014/03/caffeine-murray-carpenter-energy-drink-keurig-cup-coffee

12 Easy Ways to Prepare Yummy Coffee, http://www.vijayforvictory.com/how-to/12-yummy-ways-to-prepare-coffee/3988/

Mercola, Dr, Mounting Evidence Suggests Coffee May Actually Have Therapeutic Health Benefits, http://articles.mercola.com/sites/articles/archive/2012/09/16/coffee-health-benefits.aspx

Fries E, Detterboom L, Kirschbaum C, The Cortisol Awakening Response (CAR): Facts and Future Directions, http://www.ncbi.nlm.nih.gov/pubmed/18854200

Chapter 4

Clare, Cassandra, Quotes About Coffee, http://www.goodreads.com/quotes/tag/coffee

Gray, Richard, Best Time to Drink a Cup of Coffee: 10.30am, http://
www.telegraph.co.uk/news/newstopics/howaboutthat/10430303/Best-
time-to-drink-a-cup-of-coffee-10.30am.html

Warner, Jennifer, How to Drink Coffee, http://www.webmd.com/food-
recipes/features/how-to-drink-coffee

Hannum. Clair, Science Figured Out the Best Times of Day to Drink
Coffee, http://www.thefrisky.com/2013-11-13/science-figured-out-the-
best-times-of-day-to-drink-coffee/

The Best Time for Your Coffee, http://neurosciencedc.blogspot.
com/2013/10/the-best-time-for-your-coffee.html

Clark, Nancy, The Facts About Caffeine and Athletic Performance,
http://www.active.com/articles/the-facts-about-caffeine-and-athletic-
performance

Smith, Michael, Allen, Coffee Blending for the Home Roaster, http://
www.ineedcoffee.com/08/coffee-blending/

Medicines in My Home: Caffeine and Your Body, http://
www.fda.gov/downloads/drugs/resourcesforyou/consumers/
buyingusingmedicinesafely/understandingover-the-countermedicines/
ucm205286.pdf

Purdy, Kevin, What Caffeine Actually Does to Your Brain, http://
lifehacker.com/5585217/what-caffeine-actually-does-to-your-brain

50 Ways Caffeine Effects the Human Body,

http://arealfoodlover.wordpress.com/2012/03/20/50-ways-caffeine-
effects-the-human-body/

Wurtman, Judith, PhD, Can You Caffeinate Yourself to a Lower Weight?
http://www.huffingtonpost.com/judith-j-wurtman-phd/caffeine-weight-
loss_b_1846721.html

Caffeine Safe Limits: How to Determine Your Safe Daily Dose, http://
www.caffeineinformer.com/caffeine-safe-limits

Tarantola, Andrew, How Much Coffee Is Too Much? http://gizmodo.
com/how-much-coffee-is-too-much-1538715954

Caffeine, http://www.dorchesterhealth.org/caffeine.htm

What Happens in Your Body, After Drinking Coffee, http://www.coffeelab.nl/blog/128/www.coffeelab.nl.html

Godoy, Maria, How Many Cups of Coffee Per Day Are Too Many? http://www.npr.org/blogs/thesalt/2013/08/17/212710767/how-many-cups-of-coffee-per-day-is-too-many

Mc Laughlin, Angus, Is Caffeine an Appetite Suppressant? http://www.livestrong.com/article/480188-is-caffeine-an-appetite-suppressant/

Isacks, Kathy, Caffeine's Effect on Hunger, Suppressant or Stimulant? http://www.mynetdiary.com/caffeines-effect-on-hunger-suppressant-or.html

Abbate, Emily, 5 Appetite Suppressants That'll Help You Lose Unwanted Pounds, http://thestir.cafemom.com/healthy_living/152725/5_appetite_suppressants_thatll_help

What Is Caffeine?, https://studentaffairs.duke.edu/studenthealth/nutrition/nutrition-resources-information/caffeine

Chapter 5

Mackintosh, James, Quotes About Coffee, http://www.goodreads.com/quotes/tag/coffee?page=2

Klein, Sarah, 12 Surprising Sources of Caffeine, http://magazine.foxnews.com/food-wellness/12-surprising-sources-caffeine

Is There Caffeine in Beers Brewed With Coffee? http://www.beeradvocate.com/community/threads/is-there-caffeine-in-beers-brewed-with-coffee.48083/

Shy, Leta, How Much Soda Do You Drink a Day? http://www.fitsugar.com/How-Much-Soda-Do-Americans-Drink-Day-24154125

Caffeine in Food, http://www.caffeineinformer.com/caffeine-in-candy

Foods Highest in Caffeine, http://nutritiondata.self.com/foods-00013100000000000000-1.html?

Krummel DA, Seligson FH, Guthrie HA, Hyperactivity: Is Candy Causal? http://www.ncbi.nlm.nih.gov/pubmed/8747098

Belsky, Gail, Caffeine and Sugar: Why These Energy Boosters

Are Poor Substitutes for Sleep, http://www.health.com/health/article/0,,20411476,00.html

Reason, Jerri Ann, Effects of Caffeine and Sugar, http://www.livestrong.com/article/85251-effects-caffeine-sugar/

Brownlee, Christen, Caffeine Gives a Small Boost to Painkillers, http://www.cfah.org/hbns/2012/caffeine-gives-a-small-boost-to-painkillers-effectiveness

Controlling Pain With Caffeine, http://worldofcaffeine.com/controlling-pain/

Pain Reliever Plus (Acetaminophen, Aspirin and Caffeine) Tablet, Film Coated, http://dailymed.nlm.nih.gov/dailymed/lookup.cfm?setid=8c1fd4b1-c62a-438f-a4ce-8734187c34a1

Caffeine in Drinks, http://www.caffeineinformer.com/caffeine-content/rockstar-energy-water

Chiang, Austin, MD, Buzzed Kids Switching From Soda to Energy Drinks, http://abcnews.go.com/blogs/health/2014/02/10/buzzed-kids-switching-from-soda-to-energy-drinks/

Uberlacker, Sheryl, Energy Drinks Linked to Depression, Substance Abuse in Teens: Study, http://www.ctvnews.ca/health/energy-drinks-linked-to-depression-substance-abuse-in-teens-study-1.1717569

Quirk, Mary Beth, Forget Energy Drinks – New Study Says Kids Are Downing More Coffee Than Before, http://consumerist.com/2014/02/11/forget-energy-drinks-new-study-says-kids-are-downing-more-coffee-than-before/

Lippincott, Williams, Wilkins, Wolters Kluwer Health, Teens Who Consume Energy Drinks More Likely to Use Alcohol, Drugs, http://www.sciencedaily.com/releases/2014/02/140204111804.htm

Did You Know? http://energydrink.redbull.com/amount-of-caffeine-in-red-bull

DeNoon, Daniel J, How Much Caffeine Is in Your Energy Drink? http://www.webmd.com/food-recipes/news/20121025/how-much-caffeine-energy-drink

Schocker, Laura, 10 Things You Might Know About Caffeine, http://www.huffingtonpost.com/2013/08/25/caffeine-facts_n_3814825.html

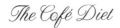

Mayo Clinic Staff, How Much Is Too Much? http://www.mayoclinic.org/healthy-living/nutrition-and-healthy-eating/in-depth/caffeine/art-20045678

Chapter 6

Lynch, David, Coffee Quotes, http://www.brainyquote.com/quotes/keywords/coffee_2.html

Digestive Statistics for the United States, http://digestive.niddk.nih.gov/statistics/statistics.aspx

Physiol, Am J, Nutrient Tasting and Signaling Mechanisms in the Gut. 11. The Intestine as a Sensory Organ: Neural, Endocrine, and Immune Responses, http://www.ncbi.nlm.nih.gov/pubmed/10564096

The Beginner's Guide to Intermittent Fasting, http://www.nerdfitness.com/blog/2013/08/06/a-beginners-guide-to-intermittent-fasting/

Creating S.M.A.R.T. Goals, http://topachievement.com/smart.html

Chapter 7

Coffee Quotes, http://www.brainyquote.com/quotes/keywords/coffee_2.html

O'Brien, Mary, Is Coffee the New Wine? http://www.smh.com.au/entertainment/restaurants-and-bars/is-coffee-the-new-wine-20101115-17u1l.html

Perez, Irene C, You Can Pair Coffee With Good Meal and Wine, http://lifestyle.inquirer.net/26115/you-can-pair-coffee-with-good-meal-and-wine

Macrae, Fiona, Why Eggs for Breakfast Will Keep Those Hunger Pangs Away Until Lunchtime, http://www.dailymail.co.uk/health/article-2143181/Why-eggs-breakfast-hunger-pangs-away-lunchtime.html

Goodwin, Lindsey, Coffee Pairings, http://coffeetea.about.com/od/foodmeetsdrinks/a/ClassicCoffeePairings.htm

The Art of Balancing Coffee With Breakfast, http://www.upstart.net.au/2010/02/10/the-art-of-balancing-coffee-with-breakfast/

Tallmadge, Katherine, Eggs Don't Deserve Their Bad Reputation, Studies Show (Op-Ed), http://www.livescience.com/39353-eggs-dont-deserve-bad-reputation.html

Pairing Food With Coffee, http://www.tastemag.co.za/Hottopics-461/Pairing-food-with-coffee.aspx

Chapter 8

Emden, Lorenzo, The Caffeinated Quotes Compendium, http://www.coffeeconfidential.org/history/coffee-quotes/

Coffee Pairing, http://allrecipes.com/howto/coffee-pairing/

Coffee And Food Pairing Dinner, http://www.home-barista.com/knockbox/coffee-and-food-pairing-dinner-t26339.html

Schulman, Jim, Ultra-Lite Roasts For Food-Coffee Pairings, http://www.coffeed.com/viewtopic.php?f=21&t=2148

Italian Food Rules – No Cappuccino After 10am, http://tuscantraveler.com/2011/florence/italian-food-rules-no-cappuccino-after-10am/

Coffee With Your Dinner, http://www.100miles.com/coffee-with-your-dinner/

How to Drink Coffee Like the French, http://goutaste.com/how-to-drink-coffee-like-the-french/

University of Florida, Decaffeinated Coffee Is Not Caffeine-Free, Experts Say, http://www.sciencedaily.com/releases/2006/10/061012185602.htm

The Definitive Guide to Grains, http://www.marksdailyapple.com/definitive-guide-grains/#axzz30A2rDFJi

Kresser, Chris, Do Carbs Kill Your Brain?, http://chriskresser.com/do-carbs-kill-your-brain

Lugavere, Max, Your "Healthy" Diet Could Be Quietly Killing Your Brain, http://www.psychologytoday.com/blog/the-optimalist/201310/your-healthy-diet-could-be-quietly-killing-your-brain

Beck, Melinda, Schatz, Amy, Americans' Eating Habits Take a Healthier Turn, Study Finds, http://online.wsj.com/news/articles/SB10001424052702304149404579323092916490748

Chapter 9

Albers, Susan, The10 Best Healthy Eating Quotes, http://www.psychologytoday.com/blog/comfort-cravings/201107/the-10-best-healthy-eating-quotes

Girdwain, Jessica, 15 Terrible Snacks for Weight Loss, http://www.prevention.com/weight-loss/weight-loss-tips/15-worst-snacks-weight-loss?s=16

Goodwin Artis, Elizabeth, The Worst Snacks for Your Body, http://www.huffingtonpost.com/2012/08/09/worst-snacks-for-body_n_1760945.html

Worst Snack Foods, http://www.livestrong.com/article/379461-worst-snack-foods/

Zizza CA, Arsiwalla DD, Ellison KJ, Contribution Of Snacking To Older Adults' Vitamin, Carotenoid, and Mineral Intakes, http://www.ncbi.nlm.nih.gov/pubmed/20430139

Paleo Grubs, 53 Healthy Paleo Snacks to Keep You Satisfied Between Meals, http://paleogrubs.com/healthy-snacks

Caloric Restriction, http://www.lef.org/protocols/lifestyle_longevity/caloric_restriction_01.htm

Foods for Dunking: Best Food and Beverage Combos, http://www.thekitchn.com/foods-for-dunking-best-food-an-78961

Top 5 Coffee Snacks, http://www.vanhoutte.com/en-ca/c-the-coffee-blog/coffee-culture/topsnacks

Top 28 Best Healthy Snacks, http://www.womenshealthmag.com/weight-loss/100-calorie-snacks

Chapter 10

Morrow, Nate, 10 Inspiring Quotes for Exercise Motivation This Fall, http://www.huffingtonpost.com/builtlean/exercise-quotes_b_3929821.html

Mental Performance, http://www.coffeeandhealth.org/research-centre/overview/caffeine-and-mental-alertness/

Bailey, Chris, How to Get as Much Energy out of Caffeine as Possible, http://ayearofproductivity.com/get-more-energy-out-of-caffeine/

Lee, Kevin, The Science of Motivation: Your Brain on Dopamine, http://blog.idonethis.com/post/70179626669/the-science-of-motivation-your-brain-on-dopamine

How Caffeine Effects Your Mood, http://glasgowspcmh.org.uk/information/health/caffeine.php

DiSalvo, David, What Caffeine Really Does to Your Brain, http://www.forbes.com/sites/daviddisalvo/2012/07/26/what-caffeine-really-does-to-your-brain/

Dr, Wenk, Gary, Why Does Coffee Make Us Feel So Good?, http://www.psychologytoday.com/blog/your-brain-food/201110/why-does-coffee-make-us-feel-so-good

Downey, Roger, Health: Does Coffee Make You Feel Sleepy?, http://www.chicagoreader.com/chicago/how-does-caffeine-affect-nervous-system-health-research/Content?oid=875717

Tackett, Rachel, Coffee Makes You Sleepy! Nutritionist Explains The Surprising Truth About Caffeine, http://en.rocketnews24.com/2013/06/11/coffee-makes-you-sleepy-nutritionist-explains-the-surprising-truth-about-caffeine/

McCoy, William, The Effect of Caffeine on Bowel Movement, http://www.livestrong.com/article/414580-the-effects-of-caffeine-on-bowel-movements/

Chapter 11

Morrow, Nate, 10 Inspiring Quotes for Exercise Motivation This Fall, http://www.huffingtonpost.com/builtlean/exercise-quotes_b_3929821.html

Santos, Victor, Santos, Vander, Caffeine Reduces Reaction Time and Improves Performance in Simulated-Contest of Taekwondo, http://www.ncbi.nlm.nih.gov/pmc/articles/PMC3942723/

Wortman, Joshua, Caffeine Enhances Muscle Performance, http://breakingmuscle.com/nutrition/caffeine-enhances-muscle-performance

Olsen, Kelly, The Effects of Caffeine on Exercise Performance, https://www.weightlossresources.co.uk/exercise/workouts/caffeine-performance.htm

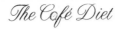

Graham, TE, Caffeine and Exercise: Metabolism, Endurance and Performance, http://www.ncbi.nlm.nih.gov/pubmed/11583104

GL, Warren, Effect of Caffeine Ingestion on Muscular Strength and Endurance: A Meta-Analysis, http://www.ncbi.nlm.nih.gov/pubmed/20019636

Krupa, Donna, Post-Exercise Caffeine Helps Muscles Refuel, http://www.the-aps.org/mm/hp/Audiences/Public-Press/For-the-Press/releases/Archive/08/24.html

Laurent, Didier, Schnieder, Kevin, Effects of Caffeine on Muscle Glycogen Utilization and the Neuroendocrine Axis During Exercise, http://press.endocrine.org/doi/full/10.1210/jcem.85.6.6655

Aubrey, Allison, Coffee: A Little Really Does Go a Long Way, http://www.npr.org/templates/story/story.php?storyId=6155178

Riggio, Gina, How Long Does the Caffeine From Coffee Stay in Your System, http://www.livestrong.com/article/272782-how-long-does-coffee-caffeine-stay-in-your-system/

Issa, Parker, Crush Your Workouts With Coffee, http://www.mensfitness.com/nutrition/what-to-drink/crush-your-workouts-with-coffee

Dr Roussell, Mike, Ask the Diet Doctor: The Workout Benefits of Coffee, http://www.shape.com/healthy-eating/diet-tips/ask-diet-doctor-workout-benefits-coffee

Reynolds, Gretchen, How Coffee Can Galvanize Your Workout, http://well.blogs.nytimes.com/2011/12/14/how-coffee-can-galvanize-your-workout/?_php=true&_type=blogs&_r=0

Chapter 12

400 Motivational Weight Loss Quotes, http://www.fitnessforweightloss.com/helpful-weight-loss-quotes/

Highest Rated Coffees, https://www.coffeereview.com/allreviews.cfm?search=1

Top 5 Most Expensive Coffee Beans, http://www.walltowatch.com/view/2778/Top+5+most+expensive+coffee+beans

10 Weird Facts About Coffee, http://www.rd.com/slideshows/10-weird-facts-about-coffee#slideshow=slide20

17 Fun Facts About Coffee: Some Weird, Interesting, Untold Coffee-Facts, http://coffeeloversunited.com/17-fun-facts-about-coffee-some-weird-interesting-untold-coffee-facts/

20 Awesome Facts About Coffee, http://likes.com/misc/12-awesome-facts-about-coffee?page=15

Gunnars, Kris, Top 13 Evidence-Based Health Benefits of Coffee, http://authoritynutrition.com/top-13-evidence-based-health-benefits-of-coffee/

Van Dam, Rob, Coffee Consumption and Risk of Type 2 Diabetes Mellitus, http://www.sciencedirect.com/science/article/pii/S014067360211436X

Consuming Coffee Before Working Out, http://www.fitday.com/fitness-articles/fitness/weight-loss/consuming-caffeine-before-working-out.html#b

Dr Graham, Terry, SSE #60: Caffeine and Exercise Performance, http://www.gssiweb.org/Article/sse-60-caffeine-and-exercise-performance

Caffeine and Exercise Performance, http://www.acsm.org/docs/current-comments/caffeineandexercise.pdf

About the Author

Béla Csepregi was not always a coffee aficionado and enthusiast. Born in Hungary, he earned his college degree as a Human Resource Specialist and worked with the Hungarian government until all that changed just about a decade ago when Csepregi and his family relocated to the U.S.

A few years after the migration, he started working in the coffee industry and almost immediately his new profession became his passion. Csepregi became fascinated by the roasting process and blending different types to create new flavors. It became like a form of art for him. He also happened to notice a happy accidental side effect, *appetite suppression*. This inspired Csepregi to do extensive research and take it a step further—develop a diet plan based on his findings.

In his first book, The Café Diet, he teaches readers how to utilize the power of the coffee bean to curb cravings and appetite. He also demonstrates how to improve eating habits for better health as well as impressive weight loss. Learn about the origins of a cup of Java while also discovering how to use coffee for diet and wellness. For more information on Csepregi visit, **www.thecafediet.com**

Made in the USA
San Bernardino, CA
07 June 2017